⧼RESTORATIVE⧽

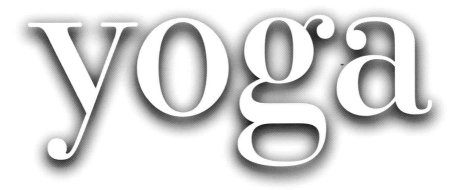

REVISED & UPDATED

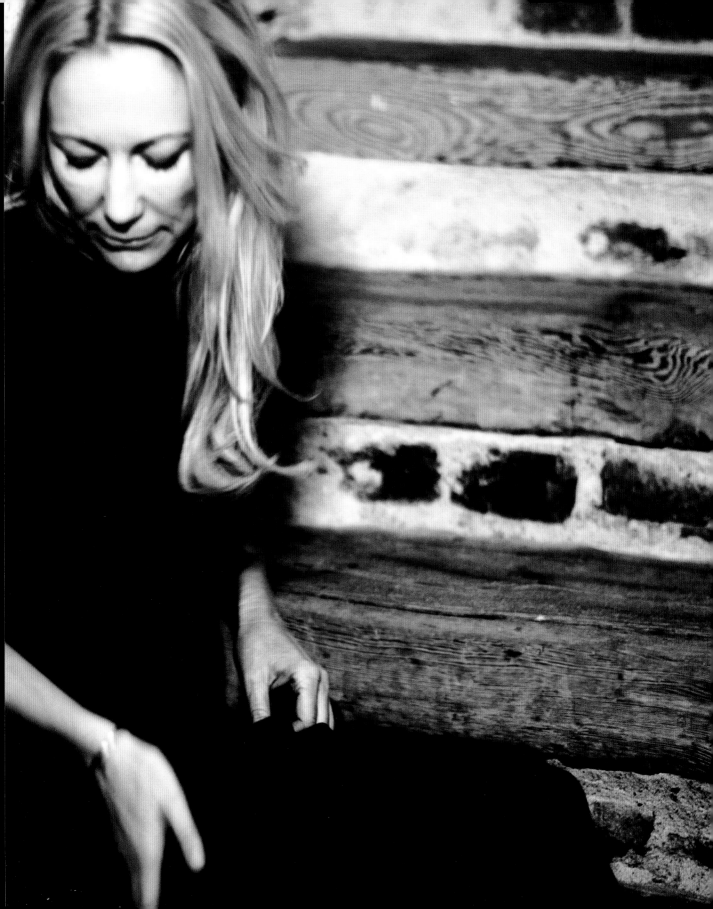

~RESTORATIVE~

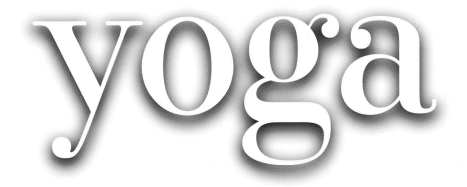
yoga

REVISED & UPDATED

REDUCE STRESS, GAIN ENERGY, AND FIND BALANCE

ULRICA NORBERG

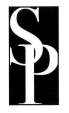

Skyhorse Publishing

Skyhorse Publishing books may be purchased in bulk at special discounts for sales promotion, corporate gifts, fund-raising, or educational purposes. Special editions can also be created to specifications. For details, contact the Special Sales Department, Skyhorse Publishing, 307 West 36th Street, 11th Floor, New York, NY 10018or info@skyhorsepublishing.com.

Skyhorse® and Skyhorse Publishing® are registered trademarks of Skyhorse Publishing, Inc.®, a Delaware corporation.

Visit our website at www.skyhorsepublishing.com.

10 9 8 7 6 5 4 3

Library of Congress Cataloging-in-Publication Data is available on file.

Cover design by Laura Klynstra
Cover photo by Sebastian Forsman

Print ISBN: 978-1-5107-0530-2

Printed in China

Important Note:
If you are unsure regarding your health status or if you have any imbalances you might think are affected through yoga practice, please seek advice from a doctor or professional physical therapist before embarking on this practice. This book is by no means a substitute to an experienced yoga teacher who can see your needs and can support you in your practice.

TABLE OF CONTENTS

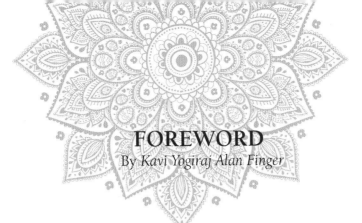

FOREWORD
By Kavi Yogiraj Alan Finger

It is with utmost pleasure that I am recommending this book to whomever is interested in personal growth, therapeutics, spirituality, science, yoga, meditation, or just in enhancing one's health.

There are so many books on yoga out there today, but few are written by someone like Ulrica who fully understands the depths and science of yoga, and who is equally well-trained academically.

This book is one of a kind—generous, sincere, and wise, like Ulrica. It shows the importance of pausing and reflection and how we can integrate this art into our living. Ulrica also focuses on the intimate relationship between science and spirituality and what this beautiful connection can do for us as individuals as well for humanity as a whole.

One of the great teachings of yoga is called *Kaivalya,* which in Sanskrit means "space from the mind." When you are not engrossed in your mind, you don't react to things, but instead you *respond.* One responds from the spirit, the source of inspiration, insight, creativity, and intuition, which are things that all humans need in this fast-paced world we live in.

The Ishta approach—developed by Mona Anand and Gina Menza, that Ulrica describes in this book—is designed to help you to develop that space in your mind, and the ability to enjoy longer periods of meditation. Meditation is the process of allowing your brain to become accustomed to stillness, which gives us the ability to gain perspective and distance, which we need in order to balance ourselves better.

It has been a privilege to be Ulrica's mentor and teacher for eight years now, and to witness her amazing growth as a yogi. When she came to me, she had already mastered so much, so I went on to teach her the science of the subtle body, which Ulrica has incorporated partly into this book.

Ulrica stands solid in the yogic tradition, honoring anyone and everything she is a part of, and she is established in the academic worlds and areas of creativity and human sciences. I am proud to have initiated her into the ISHTA lineage as a Yogiraj, Yoga Master.

Our modern society needs to de-stress and calm down mentally so that we can see life with a clearer perspective. I am confident that this book will help many to achieve that and help unlock one's hidden treasures.

Alan Finger

New York City
February 2016

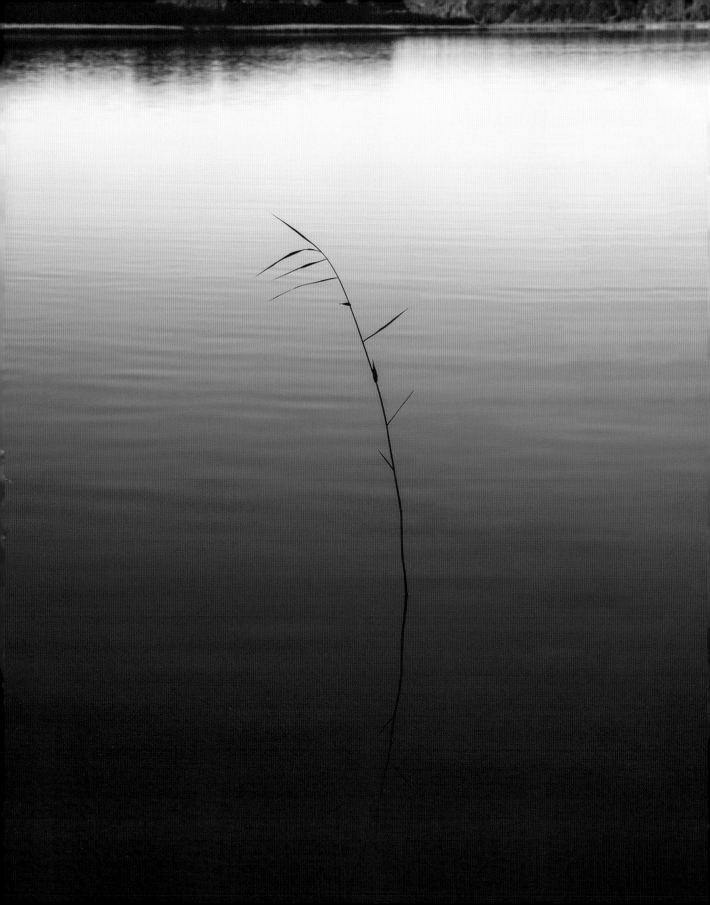

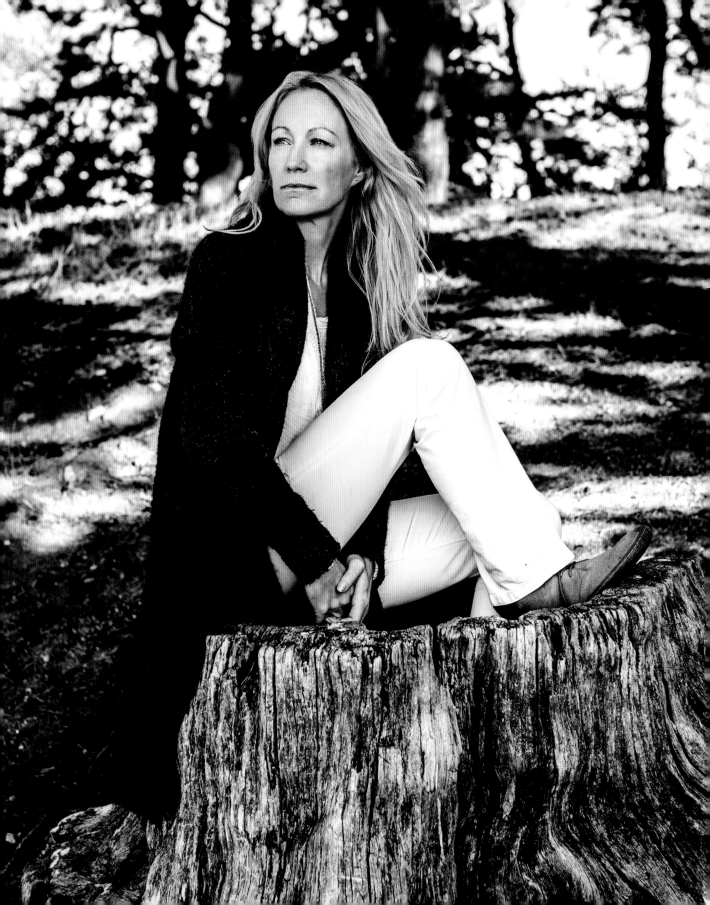

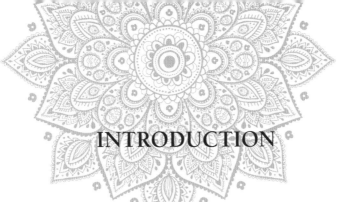

INTRODUCTION

Life and the Importance of Pausing

"The present moment is filled with joy and happiness. If you are attentive, you will see it."
—Thich Nhat Hanh

When one starts to reflect upon life and its measures, one marvels at the vastness of the whole thing. Life is fascinating, scary, beautiful, mysterious, and yet very relevant because it involves you and me and all living things in this universe. It is what connects us. Right here, right now.

Life contains and involves everything. This everything possesses many definitions. Life refers to a collective phenomenon and to the ability of an individual organism to metabolize and grow, and life refers to the history of activities that an organism undertakes. Life is also the sum of our living: one's experiences, discoveries, movement, and moments. Einstein once said that life is like riding a bicycle. In order to keep our balance, we have to keep moving, keep living.

A Buddhist thought around this is that life is movement, or change. The more fluid you are, moving with movement, the more alive you become. In yoga, life is what is experienced. Its philosophy also claims that life is being expressed in our cellular structure and it is linked together by life force: *prana*.

PRANA

We want our life force to flow uninterruptedly within our channels in order to be in homeostasis, balance. Over thousands of years, yogis have researched through their own and others' practices that the body, mind, and spirit work in correlation and in connection to one another. If our circulation of life gets stuck somewhere due to too much stress and tension, then what we need to do is to unlock the blockages of *prana* and homeostasis will return.

In yoga, we work with tension and through different techniques we wish to move deeper into it, step by step, day by day, practicing again and again, until we reach its core. Then we stay with it and use releasing techniques like slow poses, visualization, breath, and silence in order for the tension to resolve. We need to slow things down in the core of tension so the bodily systems that have perhaps been drained of energy can take some time to recover new energy, and slowly the stress and tension release their grip.

Take a sponge as an example. We leave it close to water and it will slowly start to move toward the liquid in order to absorb it. That is the code, the programming of that texture. We can look at our own systems in a similar way. The more we use them the wrong way, the more we take away from their binary code intelligence.

This idea is shared in general in medicine and, similar to yoga (though carried out in different ways), its aim is to lower the thresholds so the obstruction of flow can be reduced in order to get the blood pumping and nerves to speak with each other again. Here they use medicines, surgery, and other techniques, but with the same aim in general.

Actually, the deeper one looks into yoga and its scriptures, one realizes that much of yoga is scientific. Yogic science has always asked questions, realizing that everything is changing and everything is integrated and connected in different ways. To understand how things function, how we can understand ourselves and our race better, we need to reflect, sit with things, try out our theories, have personal experiences—to study and lift our gaze to actually get a better view.

What yoga has that modern science lacks so far are the years behind the research. Yoga has thousands of years of such research and is built upon wisdom, whereas modern science, lacking the years, makes up for some of it with technological evolution and focused research.

This book is an attempt to share some of my own findings and experience around how to decompress, de-stress, and relax into better shape. Many of us haven't been taught how to unwind and our culture is feeding us the idea that looking inside is something we shouldn't focus on, that it's lame and doesn't accomplish anything. The "being" part of being human has been lost for many people today. We are more human *doings* than human *beings*. So, as I have learned through my own journey, and what has helped me to excel beyond what I thought possible, the most important thing is the pause.

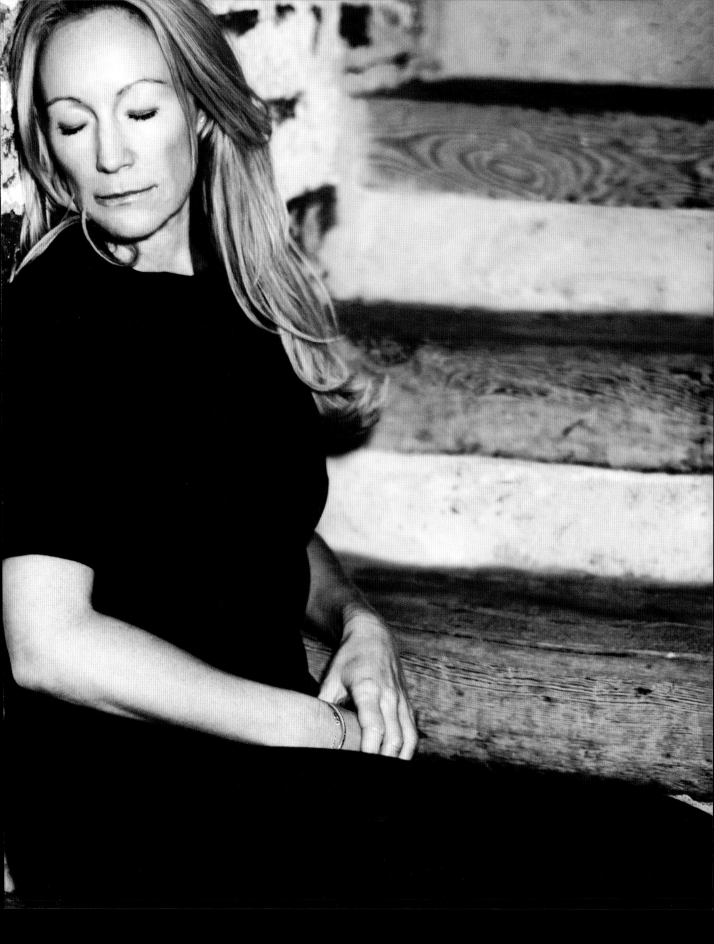

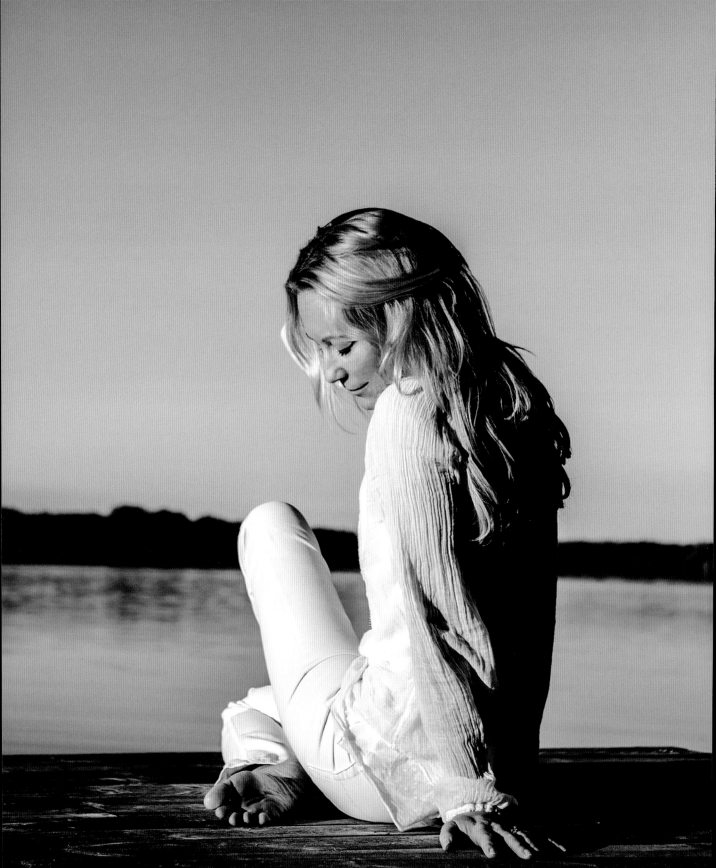

I don't believe it is weakness to slow down our lives. It is actually strength since we have taken away many natural pauses in our daily living here in the West. We live so fast today that we are starting to pay a pretty big price for that high speed, tension, and stress. We see so many new diseases that are stress related, yet our governments fall on their faces all the time, consumed by challenges in-house and globally. We seem to fight more with each other, ourselves, and life itself.

Scientists and politicians are standing still, despite mind-blowing facts about many health problems of today, and it is costing too much money for our societies. Our way of living is writing checks our bodies can't cash.

What if we took another route? What if we try something else? What if we yoked doing and being, to a much greater extent? What if some answers about the growing health problems lie in doing less rather than doing more?

Restorative yoga is a yogic approach of limiting the options for the body to continue to be carried by fear, pain, stress, and tension by using different props to make us weightless; removing all pressure on the body's joints; and holding the poses for six minutes up to an hour. Restorative yoga aids the so-called "Relaxation Response" in the brain, which is the healing mode for our being.

I will speak more on restorative yoga as a practice and how you can start benefiting from this practice in your life. In Chapter 5, I will also convey what the relaxation response is and why it is so important for our health to start to own the ability to relax and unwind, since so many of us have lost that skill.

As we move along the chapters, I hope you will see that when we yoke experimenting with wisdom, action with pausing, movement with stillness, and science with spirituality, we get a better understanding of this thing called life and how we can live more fully and in more balanced ways.

INQUIRE AND INVESTIGATE

I believe it to be true that for our practice to be successful and fruitful, to see its results in our own personal growth and also to achieve higher levels of health, we need go inward with a more inquiring and investigative approach. The way I have laid out the information in this book is not to say how you should live your life or how to do restorative yoga my way, or anyone's way. My aim is to inspire you to find your own way of doing yoga so you can live your life in better balance than before.

I will share some great things I have learned through my trainings, from my teachers, and from the practice itself in the hope of helping you to attain the tools needed to find balance. I also share my own reflections on aspects of tension-releasing and de-stressing and how we can merge through these thresholds to give our body back its powers and also to increase circulation and limit toxins and negativity.

When I first started yoga, I was introduced to a quite physical way of doing it, in which my teachers were strict and options were limited. It was good for me at the time, not to have so many options, to limit possibilities and variations in an attempt to simplify things. After a while, however, I began to feel insecure and vulnerable in my practice, so I moved on and kept searching for a yogic approach that resonated better with me. Years passed and through many in-depth studies in various styles of yoga, my yoga practice grew and became strong and selfless. I am so utterly grateful for all the techniques I have learned and for the knowledge and wisdom I have come across through several phenomenal teachers.

It wasn't until I found a more flexible approach, in the ISHTA yoga lineage, that I really came to terms with who I was and began to deeply evolve as a yogi, teacher, and human being. The ISHTA approach resonates with me greatly since it honors all styles and paths of yoga and has a more scientific-spirituality fusion orientation, which continues to appeal to me.

This book delves into restorative yoga through an ISHTA lens, which means that we look at individuality and adaptation in greater length and depth. I was first introduced to the ISHTA approach to restorative yoga in Mona Anand and Gina Menza's Restorative Training at ISHTA Yoga, now known as the Anand Menza Restorative Training.

In teaching yoga, I am deeply imbedded in the various aspects of the architecture of this practice and I acknowledge the importance of tradition. I try to help my students to evolve and find the keys of the practice by helping them get inside themselves through investigation and inquiry, since it is only when we allow ourselves to play with concepts and ideas that we start to research possibilities, and through that we evolve.

My hope is that you, through this book, will feel inspired to start exploring, finding, acknowledging, stretching, and embracing the pauses in life. Because that's where we connect to the forces of life within ourselves. That's where we can connect the outer and inner aspects of living. It is in the pauses that you connect to the intelligence inside yourself.

I will share my own thoughts, experiences, and knowledge on the topic of how we can restore, renew, and rebalance our energies in modern life. I have also invited some of my dear colleagues and friends who happen to be some of the most experienced in their field, whether spiritualism or science, and I share their findings because their voices should be heard.

So, let's investigate the intelligence behind slowing things down and finding the pauses. It is through them your life will change for the better.

Om Shanti,

Ulrica

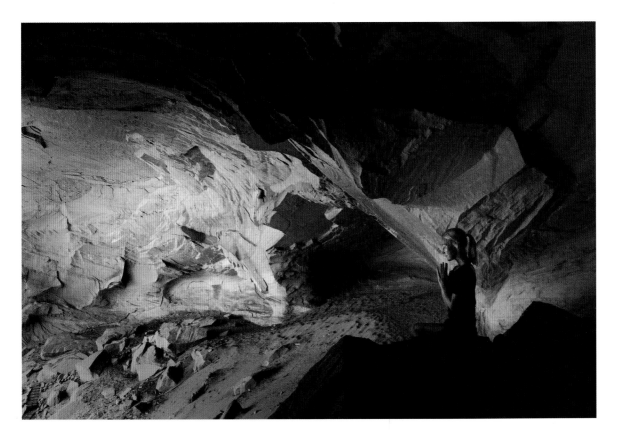

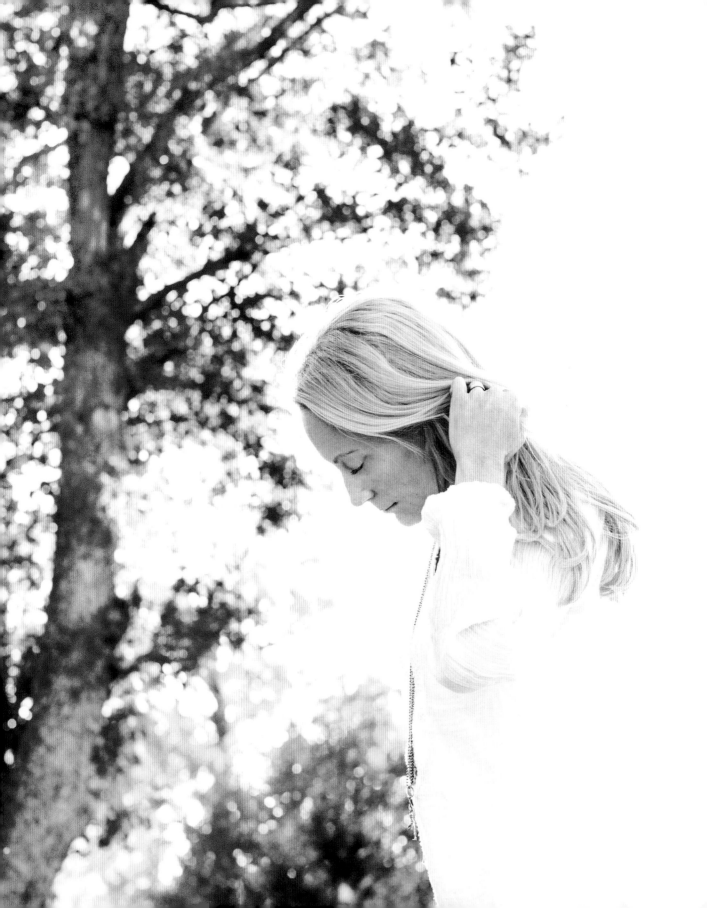

Chapter One
THE POWER OF SLOWING DOWN

"In the attitude of silence the soul finds the path in a clearer light, and what is elusive and deceptive resolves itself into crystal clearness."
—Mahatma Gandhi

Our busy minds have taken over, and our lives are being built on strenuous efforts rather than allowing them to emerge naturally and effortlessly. We might strive for more wealth but we keep feeding cultural poverty—thus, we think we are doing more but feel like we are doing nothing. Many don't know how to take a break, and many of us believe pausing is a sign of weakness.

Often we get so caught up in what everyone else is doing and what's trendy that we get lost in the excitement of the new and its pressures and we forget how to slow down and reflect upon what we are bringing into our minds and into our lives, what we allow to consume us. Or worse, we become robotic and aimlessly live our lives trying to keep up with everyone else and becoming numb to our true desires and needs.

We need to feed both our superpowers within: the "doing" mode and "being" mode. The ancient yogis understood that when they called this practice yoga, to yoke polarities. When we connect our polarities, we start connecting to our inner shrine of intelligence. There are countless reasons why it's great to keep up with the latest trends and to streamline processes in your life. It drives our productivity and frees up time to do things that are important to us, and it helps us grow. However, there are also reasons why slowing down regularly is one of the great super powers we have within.

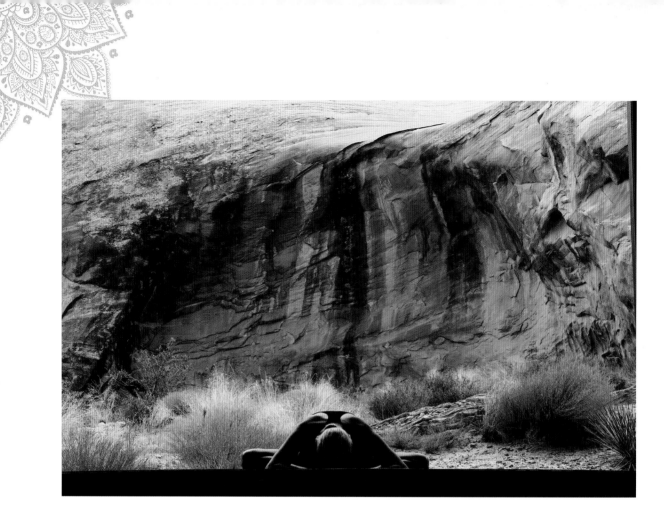

Slow and Steady Wins the Race

In the fable, "The Tortoise and the Hare," consistency and tenacity prevails over speed. This is especially true when it comes to anything worthwhile in life, anything important that you're committed to for the long haul. When you are focused on doing one thing at a time and giving it your undivided attention, you give yourself space and time to reflect and react without distraction. With a calm mind, you are less likely to feel overwhelmed and are able to tune in to your surroundings. Being focused and intentional heightens your senses and intuition and allows you to enjoy the flavors of life while making confident decisions with mental clarity and deliberate intention.

When giving attention to one object or process, you are building a strong platform and connection to create the value and trust to sustain the outcome you seek. When you slow down you embrace the "less is more" philosophy and it can go a long way. That being said,

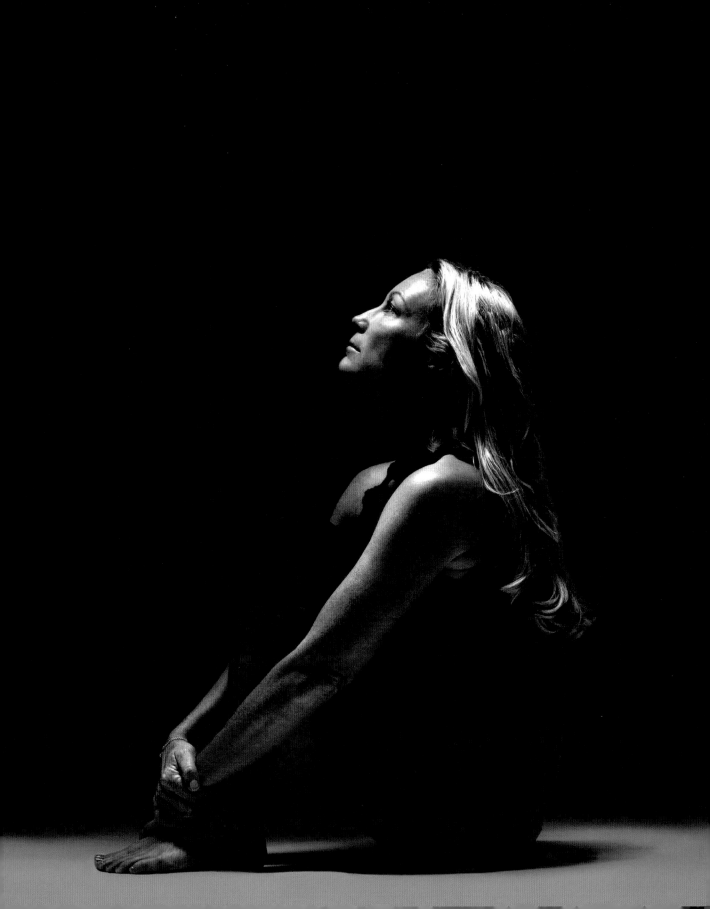

there is value in multitasking, up to a point. It helps us step up our game, forcing us to try new things and discover new ways to do things, and certain processes can actually feed each other. But it is through regular rest that one frees up the mental capital to be able to stay present and thus perform better with better resources.

Restorative Yoga

The word yoga means "to yoke." A yoga practice is meant to fuse together opposites in order to attain balance, or equanimity. In life as well as in yoga, we want to add what is not there, to find better balance. So if we are stressed, rushed, and on-the-go, we need to add in more relaxation, pausing and doing less, in order to get ourselves back into flowing better with life.

Yoga practices are designed to help an individual feel whole, so taking a yoga class can do wonders for the body, mind, and spirit. And very often when one comes into a yoga class, there are mainly physical poses, *asana*, and breathing techniques, *pranayama*, ending in the *savasana* relaxation pose for a couple of minutes; not much time is given to restore more deeply.

Yoga Master B. K. S. Iyengar developed the practice of restorative yoga. He is recognized as one of the greatest master yogis in postmodern times and is the founder of the more alignment-oriented hatha yoga style called Iyengar yoga. Iyengar learned yoga from his master and father-in-law, Sri Krishnamacharya, one of the most influential yoga masters in the twentieth century.

Iyengar learned early on while teaching yoga that pain or injury often resulted from a student straining in a pose. So he followed advice from his teacher to modify the poses, and in doing so, he got experimental and invented props out of strings, trees, bricks, rolled up blankets, and sacks of sand. He saw that modifying the poses and adding the props helped his students to move more safely into the poses and their breath improved dramatically when the alignment of the body was in better balance. He also started to see that placing students in passive poses, where the props gave the shape to the body and where the body could lean onto them, gave remarkable results in stress reduction and healing. Those of us who have had the privilege to study with him found that while he could be very strict and quite harsh, he taught us much about ourselves and the human body and how to access it in intelligent ways. Thanks to B. K. S. Iyengar, we have many phenomenal methods to heal, restore, de-stress, and reboot our systems.

As I see it, Iyengar was one of the most important teachers, since he emphasized that the body holds a deep intelligence. He was able to decode some of the mysteries of the human body and make yoga applicable to different physical conditions. I remember him saying in class once, "Go inside gently and stay. If you suffer in the pose, you need to make the pose work better for you. While you are there, experience the pose. Listen to your body, not the mind, since it bears no real truth, only reaction." His words were so important to me then and they still echo in my practice to this day.

Restorative yoga is a kind of active relaxation, since its techniques help us learn how to unwind, relax, and de-stress in order to reboot and restore our nervous system by taking as much pressure off our bodily functions as possible. The aim is to feel weightless. The way we do that is by using different props to support the body so we can let go of all tension. We stay in the poses for a long time so the nervous system will alternate from firing from its active part to its more restorative part.

So the aim is to communicate with the brain through the supported poses in a way that tells the body there is no tension, no danger anywhere. After a while, the brain gets the message and will lower the stress hormones and increase the life-enhancing hormones that we need in order to heal and feel well.

Restorative yoga is pretty clear: grab the props you need, set yourself up in a nice space, settle into a pose, stay there, let go, and breathe. Gina Menza feels, "Unlike other exercises, this practice places minimal metabolic demand on you and increases your energy rather than subtracting from it."

All the organ systems of the body benefit from deep relaxation, and a few of the measurable results are the reduction of blood pressure, serum triglycerides, and blood sugar levels, and increase of the "good cholesterol" levels. Deep relaxation also provides an improvement in digestion, fertility, elimination, the reduction of muscle tension, insomnia, and generalized fatigue.

"Restorative yoga helps to release tension on a physical, mental, and emotional level. Since our bodies store all our past experiences, when we let go of the hold on the physical body we often have strong emotional releases as suppressed emotions bubble up. For this reason, it's very important to create a supportive environment," according to Yogaraj Mona Anand, co-creator of ISHTA's approach to restorative yoga. Very often, students come into restorative on overdrive, she says. "Music, candlelight, essential oils, and gentle *asana* can help slow down their energy in preparation for restorative postures. When students have trouble surrendering, visualizations, breath awareness, and body scans are useful tools to help still the mind," she continues.

According to Mona, restorative postures are a powerful way of rebalancing our energy. "We can choose from a variety of poses to help achieve this: backbends lift our energy, forward bends calm our energy, twists calm the nervous system and help with digestion, and inversions quiet the mind. Restorative yoga can be practiced by everyone. Pillows, blocks, blankets, towels—anything that helps support the body can be used to create a restorative pose. People who aren't physically able to practice *asana*, such as the elderly and physically challenged, can practice restorative yoga and reap the benefits of deep relaxation and energy rebalancing," she adds.

This is a practice that can be done safely at home, but since poses are held for an extended period of time, a basic understanding of the practice is important initially. Or consult an experienced teacher. I learned through Mona and Gina, my dear friends and colleagues in restorative yoga, that holding postures for an extended period of time, when not correctly aligned, can lead to physical and energetic imbalances. According to Mona, there are also poses that are not appropriate for different physical and emotional issues. For example, she says, "A person with a heart condition might not want to practice an inversion, a person with lower back sensitivity may need to modify a restorative forward bend, and someone with an anxiety disorder may need to modify a backbend." So, with an understanding of the alignment of restorative postures and the benefits and contraindications of the poses we put ourselves in, you can start to explore this on your own and make it a home practice.

The first time I tried restorative yoga was in the late nineties in a class with Judith Hanson Lasater, physical therapist, Iyengar yoga teacher, and one of the most influential restorative yoga teachers today. At the time, my practice was flavored with more vigorous styles of yoga (*ashtanga*, *vinyasa*, and power yoga), but I had gotten more and more interested in the Iyengar yoga system due to its more anatomical focus and emphasis on alignment.

I heard of Judith through another Iyengar teacher I had the privilege to study with, Patricia Walden. She mentioned Judith and, when a workshop opportunity came up, I signed up, not really knowing what to expect. In the weeks leading up to her workshop, my life was chaos and I had some tough challenges, was recovering from a bad breakup, and also feeling quite lost in life.

The first day of the workshop I just wanted to run away, to get the hell out of there. My mind was so restless, my body was tensed up, and I was irritated at everyone around me. I can still hear Judith's words play back to me: pause, just be, let go. I felt so alone, vulnerable, open. I was afraid that I wouldn't be able to pick myself up after letting it all go. My controlled behavior had me in such a tight grip. I saw it, but I didn't know how to get out of it. I cried myself to sleep that night.

After the second day's first practice, it all changed. In one of the inversion poses we held for over twenty minutes, I just surrendered all of a sudden. In my mind, I heard: *Ulrica, you are here now. Do as she says. Try it out. What do you have to lose? Let the practice take care of you. You know it will. You can do it. If you break, you break. But what if you don't? What if you can heal?*

I let go and cried. An assistant came over and placed more blankets on me. She said nothing, just placed her hands gently on my shoulders and stayed there until I had no more tears. I took a couple of breaths and that was that. I got out of the pose and moved on to the next one. I felt relieved, lighter, but quite shaky.

It was like a thick armor of tension and stress I had been carrying inside for a long time was gone. That inspired me, since it felt so great. After that class, the assistant (who is now one of my closest friends) gave me a spontaneous hug and said, "Great job. That stuff needed to be released. Congratulations."

The days to follow taught me so much about myself since I took the time to focus internally. I felt safe, nurtured, held, and like I was floating—I felt free. And most importantly, I learned what relaxation was and how to get there.

Years would pass until I took a longer restorative training, and even longer before I started to teach it. I felt I still had so much to learn, so much to shed before I could settle in that seat of comfort inside myself. A couple of slow yoga trainings later and hundreds of hours being propped up on my mat, and I have grown to love, appreciate, and deeply value this practice. Today, it is a weekly necessity. It gives me such nourishment, and I see the marvelous benefits in my colleagues and students as well.

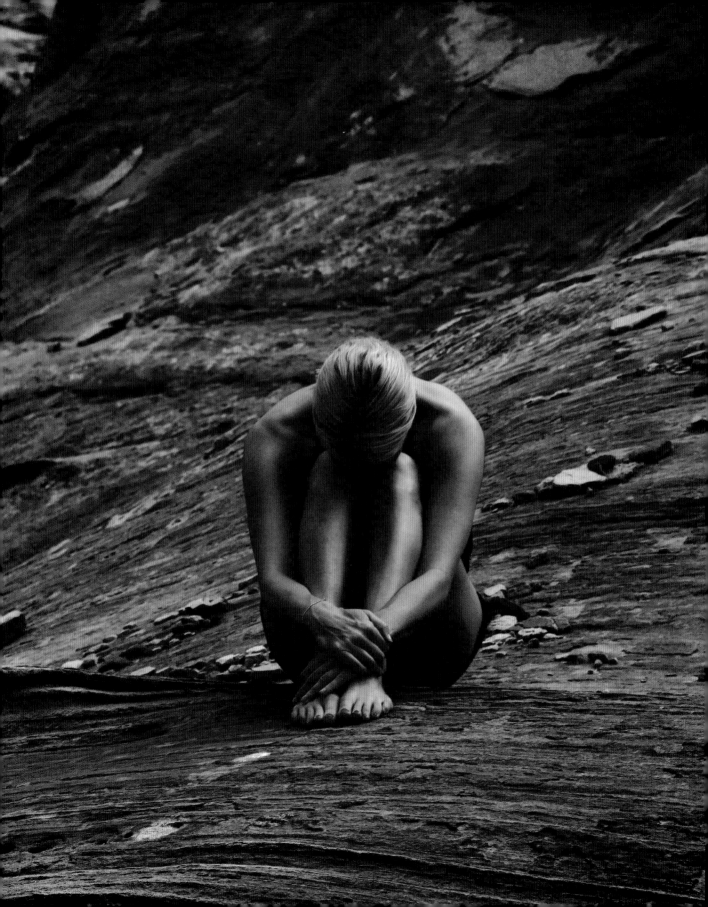

Individualizing the Practice

I share the love of this practice with two of my dear friends and yoga colleagues, Master ISHTA Teacher, Yogiraj Mona Anand and Senior ISHTA Teacher Gina Menza, who both teach restorative yoga in New York City. Together, they created the ISHTA approach to restorative yoga that stems from the Iyengar yoga method, yet adds more focus on the individualization of the practice and the subtle body. Their approach focuses on balancing physical, emotional, Ayurvedic, and energetic imbalances by integrating visualization, *pranayama*, *kriya* techniques, yoga *nidra*, and essential oils into the practice. "We teach our students to recognize their imbalances and give them the tools to bring themselves back into balance," they say in unison.

ISHTA restorative yoga brings in a more personal approach, integrating visualization, mantra, *pranayama*, and *kriya* techniques. In this way, we can teach each student to recognize their imbalances and give them the tools to find balance on their own so they can live their lives to the fullest, rather than settle for just surviving and striving. The aim is to live and appreciate life, not just survive it.

For Gina, restorative yoga balances her otherwise quite busy life since it adds relaxation, support, and stillness. For her, teaching restorative yoga is equally as divine as practicing it herself.

Gina feels that to receive the energy created by a roomful of yogis is the best gift. "Restorative yoga provides the perfect antidote to stress because it creates a supported pause," Mona says. "Softening the body, evening the breath, and quieting the mind change the actual chemistry of the body as both sides of the nervous system adjust," Gina adds.

Restorative yoga has helped Mona through severe asthma. She was continually in and out of the hospital and put on high levels of cortisone for an extended period, which created extreme anxiety and panic attacks. Practicing restorative yoga proved integral to her recovery, calming her nervous system, relaxing her body, and releasing tension from the breath, all of which had been bracing for future asthma attacks. No amount of trying to talk herself out of the situation had helped because her whole system was stuck in a heightened state of tension.

"I needed to bypass my mind and activate the parasympathetic nervous system, which is exactly what restorative does," she told me. "By completely supporting the body and being still for an extended length of time, the breath, the mind, and the nervous system begin to calm down. Different restorative poses can be used for different purposes, though they all help to calm and quiet the nervous system. There are poses that open the breath and lift our spirits when we're feeling depressed, poses that are supportive and nurturing when we're feeling anxious, and poses that target specific parts of the body where tension accumulates."

The ISHTA yoga restorative approach appeals to me greatly since it has the foundation of the Iyengar practice, yet takes it even further in ways that I can customize for my students. Through a more Tantric and Ayurvedic approach, we can aid and deepen the personal practice to reflect the seasons, age of the person, and also the individual condition, to a much greater extent. In ISHTA, we want the practice to be self-balancing—to find a yoga that resonates with the individual, a yoga that stems from what we need, not from what the mind's fluctuations tell us. And we want the practice of restorative yoga to help people to move toward meditation.

"Modern life is fast-paced and filled with stressors that contribute to a low-grade level of stress that we're often unaware of. This continuous state of sympathetic nervous system (the adrenaline-based active side of our nervous system) arousal has led to many modern day illnesses such as asthma, cancer, heart disease, and stress disorders. Restorative yoga provides the perfect antidote to stress because it creates a supported pause. By completely supporting the body and being still for extended periods, the breath, the mind, and the nervous system begin to calm," Mona says.

She continues, "Different restorative poses can be used for different purposes, though they all help to calm and quiet the nervous system. There are poses that open the breath and lift our spirits when we're feeling depressed, poses that are supportive and nurturing when we're feeling anxious, and poses that target specific parts of the body where tension accumulates. The impact restorative yoga has in releasing stress and tension is very personal." For Gina, Mona, and myself, restorative yoga has helped us through so much in our lives, and we can also witness how it has helped many of our students to achieve greater health.

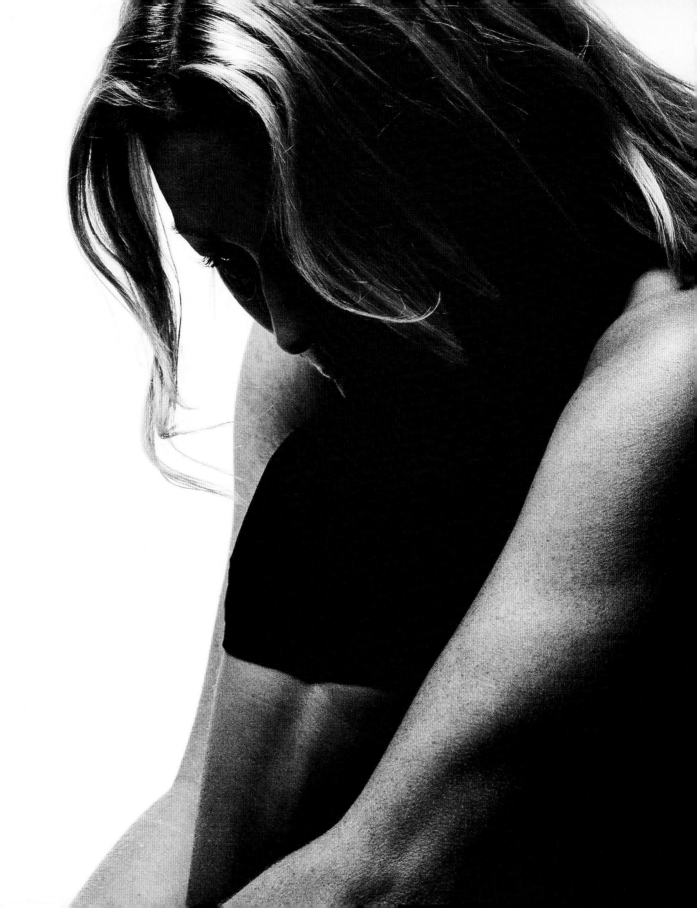

Lifeline Yoga

Restorative yoga is what I call a "lifeline" yoga practice. It helps at times when you feel weak, fatigued, stressed, before or after major life events, change of a job, divorce, through challenges in marriage, parenting, major holidays, and vacation—in any moment in life where you feel rocky, unsure, unfocused, challenged, scared, or vulnerable. And it also works beautifully as a boosting practice for athletic performance, creativity, and mood enhancement. I will elaborate further on how restorative can be used for different effects and needs later on in the book, in Chapter 5.

In 2008, my husband was diagnosed with a deadly liver condition. Since then we have almost lost him twice, but he is okay, due to great medicine and therapy. He leads a normal life today, managing a demanding and inspiring job as a process engineer (specialized in environmental water purification). Ever since that day in the summer of 2008, our life has been challenging, and the stress surrounding living with a death sentence over our heads took its toll on our relationship and marriage. One of the things that keeps us together and in balance—apart from being best friends and having the same outlook on life and shared love for our family—is that we both prioritize pauses, we reflect, and we try to live healthy. And I have seen how beneficial restorative yoga has been for him: once in a while, I put him in a pose or two. I prop him up in one pose, leave the room for twenty minutes, and come back to find him peaceful. Then I bring him into another pose and leave him again. I do that a couple of times and while he is inside these poses, I work around the house, play or talk with the kids, and attend to other things that need attention. Then we take a cup of tea and talk before bedtime. We have the best talks after our evening yoga sessions, and these talks are what glue us together and keep us running. That recipe has gotten us through many challenges over the years. And it still does.

Restorative yoga, yin yoga, *pranayama*, and meditation have all helped me tremendously in my work as a teacher and a writer, as a mother, and also in keeping myself healthy on all levels. This practice was my recovery practice a few years back when I was suffering from exhaustion, which led to depression. I was running a big yoga business, caring for my then-ill husband, taking care of our home and small children, writing and editing books, and teaching classes, workshops, and trainings. I was depleted from all the demands and expectations of me and I lost a lot of weight. I felt trapped and alone all the time, crying myself to sleep every night. I felt I had no way out.

After my doctor literally shook me and told me I had to put on the brakes, I took the last amounts of energy I had in me, and I let go of the business and some other endeavors.

I felt like such a failure. There I was: a yogi, a yoga teacher with so many tools in my belt. And yet I ended up like this. That was very humbling and totally what I needed in order to evolve and mature further as a human being. From rock bottom, I meditated, restored, and yielded my way back into balance.

For a while, I could not do anything active. Anything other than restorative, yin yoga, and gentle *pranayama*, breathing practice, would raise my heart rate too much and I would feel stressed. After months of these techniques as my sole practice, along with walks in nature on my own and with my children, I started to feel more energetic, balanced, and alive. When talking to Mona Anand about this, her words were mimicking what I was feeling: "Restorative poses supported my muscles and joints for an extended period of time, and the contraction and tension in my body began to release. This led to my nervous system firing less. Restorative poses also helped to take the tension out of my breath—since the breath is directly influenced by the state of our mind and body—and my mind started to relax and open up. This also helped my body to cleanse toxins since my circulation improved greatly, with tension releasing and a growing ability to breathe deeper and deeper. It is a two-way street—a relaxed body creates a relaxed mind and breath, and a relaxed breath and mind create a relaxed body," she so wisely shared. "Restorative yoga can calm down nervous systems, relax the body, and release tension from the mind, and it is possible to let go of the idea of stress."

Stress-Proof Your Life

We all need to stress-proof our lives. My prescription is to make yourself your number one priority. We all have twenty-four hours in a day and we can make conscious choices about how we want to spend them. Really. The majority of us can do that and have the freedom to do so. It does not have to be so complex. It is the small changes that allow great effects to emerge. It is true. Changing your life so it flows better demands very little of you.

Later on in the book, in Chapters 3 and 4, I will lay out various tips and advice on how one can reduce stress and enhance one's energies.

In my recovery from exhaustion, I had great support from my mentor Alan Finger, a counselor, great friends and family, and also from my practice. I cannot stress the importance of a practice enough. It can save lives.

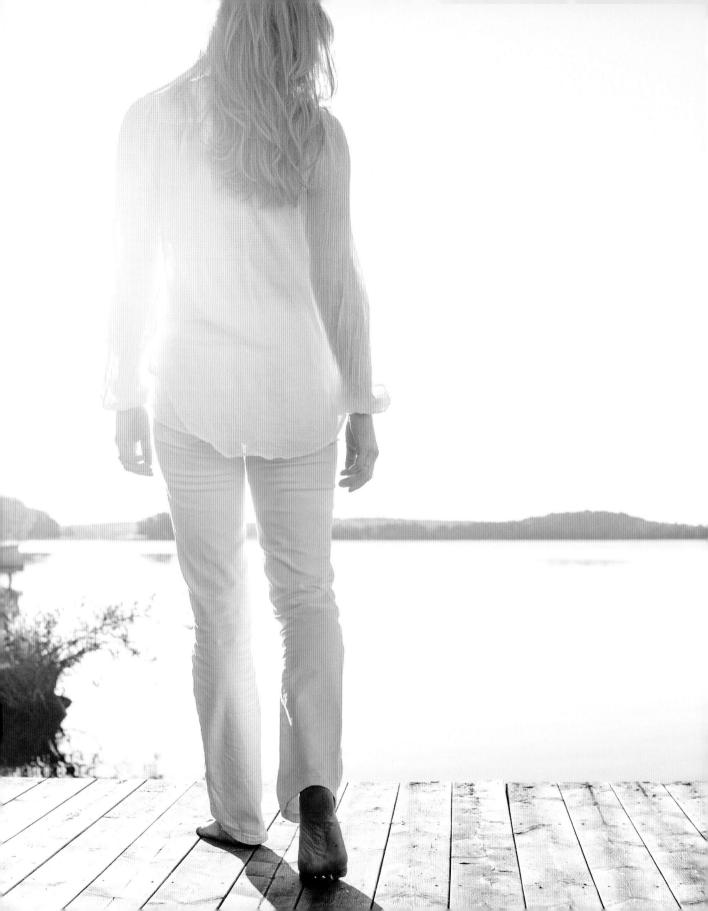

It saved me.

These days, I balance meditation and restoring techniques with more active, flowing yoga as well as walking, occasional jogging, and some gentle weight training in order to keep myself as balanced as possible. On days I don't feel like getting out of bed, I tell my mind that I don't have to. I tell myself I just have to lay on a bolster until starting the day seems like a cool idea. That process takes a couple of minutes, but I have learned that if I start by forcing myself into doing, pushing myself, I will be set back into a more depressed mindset. And the way it acts out in me is through coping and compensating. I am not my best self when in that mode. Not at all. So, I do what I can to avoid going there.

How much rest versus how much activity you need is a matter of investigation and inquiry for each and every one of us. It depends on where you are, what resources you have, and where you are coming from. A good way to measure is to reflect each day at the end of the day, see where you are and how you feel. Honestly ask yourself what you need to add in order to attain better balance. And reflect upon the answers.

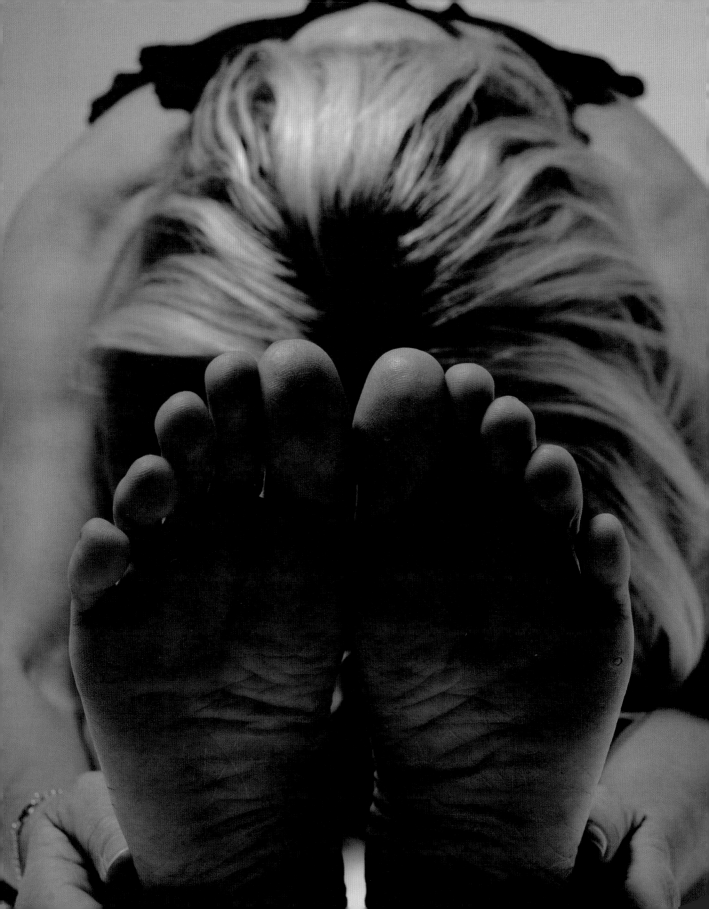

Chapter Two
THE SCIENCE BEHIND YOGA

"...ignorance is the curse of God, knowledge the wing wherewith we fly to heaven."
—William Shakespeare

Yoga only asks one question: *Who Am I?*

It's a very deep and personal question, and just by letting oneself ponder it, it grows too big to even get one's head around. This is because we try so hard to find an easy answer. We want the answer delivered to us as a sentence or a quick explanation.

As I see it, this question is more a focus, and a direction of energy. The yogic techniques are there for us to use over and over again, to adapt toward our capabilities and grow with them, finding new techniques.

I like to think of the answer to the question "who am I?" as what can be found at the top of a mountain—our own inner mountain, where the top is where we reach the understanding of who we really are. The place where we understand who we are, an embodied understanding, a sense of feeling who we are in every cell of our being. Where words are useless and thoughts superfluous.

The yogic quest, the spiritual journey, is to climb the mountain. It will take time, effort, and progression, and we have to start from the base and climb a little at a time. One step at a time.

When beginning the practice of yoga, we start with the knowledge and experience we have in that moment—and we usually become frustrated, annoyed, and disappointed. We sometimes give up, since we didn't reach the top right away or we can't see the top, so it is hard to estimate how much energy we need in order to evolve. Since the end is not visible to us, we give up or see the mountain as something we have to fight. We often get overly ambitious or intimidated, afraid, or unwilling to listen to advice from those who are wiser. We don't want to hear it takes time, since we believe we don't have time. We want the answer *now*. We just see this mountain as something to conquer, or we just let the mountain be a mountain, only there for other crazy people to climb. And we continue on, stuck in "reactive land," searching and jumping from thing to thing in the hope something is gonna give, with the mindset of *then, when, if,* and *only.* "If only I had more money, then I would do such and such," or "When I get that, then I will start doing such and such."

Or, we are stuck in that other way of living, in the alley of blame and darkness, thinking, *nothing really matters anyway, no one cares, let others do it, it is better just not to expect anything than to always get so disappointed, it was so much better before, I hate change.*

We often get caught up in the so-called "I-ness," in which we live our lives in our feelings and everything else has no real relation to life. It may sound strange, but our life is our feelings, moods, and emotions. When we are in a good mood, we are inspired by everything—the world around us, people, atmosphere, and even possessions. When we are in a bad mood, nothing can force us to feel pleased and satisfied, not even the most valuable and vital things that usually lead to happiness. When we are happy the whole world is in harmony and everything brings us joy. In other words, the meaning of life is to experience the feelings that give pleasure and joy. No matter how rich we are—in money, power, houses, cars, and sex—it means nothing if we do not appreciate and respect life's pleasures. At the same time, if we live in harmony with spirit and experience the feeling of joy and life satisfaction, we will be happy just to be alive. The meaning of life is hidden inside our emotions.

Our yoga practice should help us to live fuller lives. Our practice should help us climb a little higher every day, and if we climb too high, teach us we have to come down and rest, and next time, learn how to equalize.

We so often forget the importance of pausing, calibrating, and equalizing. We often push and go full on. So, in order to get safely up our inner mountain, we need to fail, reflect, try again, push, rest, breathe, stop, go, do, be, and mix them all up in a nice blend. That is what yoga is there to teach us: to find our own personal way, our own yoga, and our own balance where we see and connect to our fullest potential, becoming who we really are beyond all the reactions, beliefs, and fear. Yoga allows us to integrate what we already have—lots of tools inside our bodies, brains, and nervous systems. The more we yoke all of our systems together, the more they work together. For the longest time, yoga has claimed that we are self-healing creatures and that we can mend ourselves if broken. All we have to do is yoke the things we already possess: the gifts from our bodily systems. In yoga, we see that the nine systems in our bodies are connected and supposed to work in unison. When this unison is interrupted or distorted, then disease, stress, and imbalances appear.

Therefore, yoga says, let's yoke together the circuits of the systems again. These systems carry so much intelligence on their own; however, when united, we become full-powered beings that can evolve beyond the imaginary and create wonderful things.

We need to find and clear the pathways for our systems to unite. Historically, the masters of yoga tried different ways and came up with body postures, *asana*, to connect different parts of the body with other parts of the body, getting the systems (muscular system, nervous system, and skeletal system) to work and slowly find each other through doing.

The great masters understood that one system was superior in connecting all the other ones: the breathing (respiratory system), since it affected the mind and energy of the individual (endocrine system, cellular system), and in adding breathing with *asana* they saw that the overall health and balance (homeostasis) improved dramatically. They learned that a person's balance has a lot to do with how well the body circulates blood (circulatory system), since the blood carries nutrients and oxygen to all the building blocks and maintenance stations in our bodies and brains.

They started investigating how they moved, what happened when they started to breathe in different ways, or ate different things (digestion system), noting what affected them differently. After hundreds of years of exploration, inquiry, and investigation using the yogic practice, they understood that in order to reach one's ultimate potential, to understand who one is, one needs to yoke together all aspects of oneself. Over and over again. After each effort, they stopped and paused, noticing what came up, what was different, and what they could bring to the next moment. They reached the insight that in order to elevate to one's highest potential one needs not only yoking but the understanding that we are creatures that have capacities for 50 percent being and 50 percent doing within us, like the cycle of a day, like the tie with the sun and moon, the balance between light and dark, and day and night. They also learned that the polarities unite in the pauses—what modern science today explains as the micro pauses—where electrons can pass over information. Without that spaciousness between neurons, without range of mobility in our joints, without clear pathways in our arteries and veins, and without straight-on clear roads in our nervous systems, information is interrupted and we literally become confused and non-whole. By not fusing together the intelligence inside, we die faster than we should. Yogic science and its methods claim that if we want to live longer and have a great quality of life, we have to mind

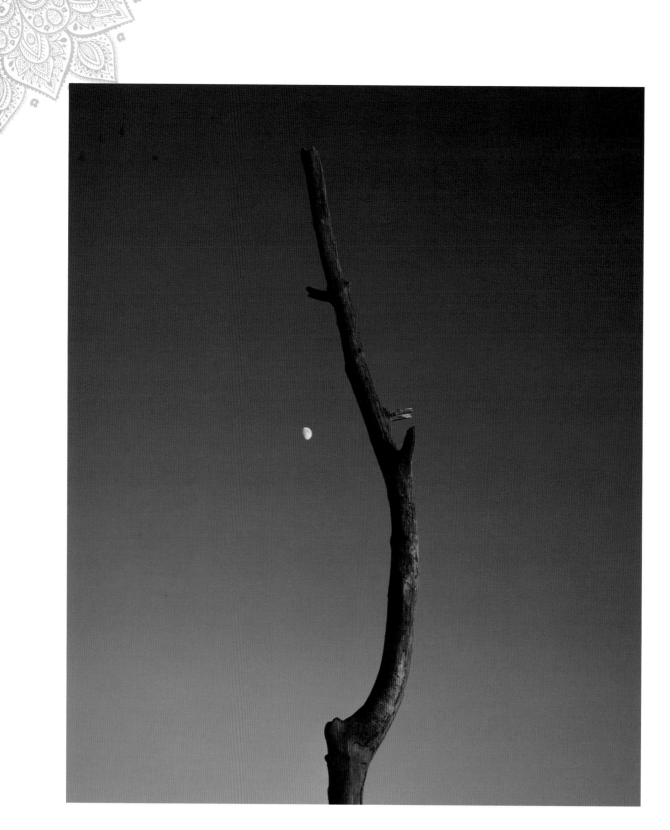

our systems and do what we can to improve their work space and make room for them to do their job. When the systems work in unison, we are in balance.

The Balancing Act

Yogic philosophy claims that we have all we need inside. All the resources are there for us to lead a great life. We have capacity and potential. It is just our stressed and imbalanced minds that tell us we don't have enough and can't do enough. This limits how we see life, and we never go up on our inner mountain to have a look out, to see our surroundings, to see our scenery, to learn about ourselves through reflection and looking at things from a distance. Stress is just a thought. If we tell ourselves we are stressed, we become stressed. Stress is not something that happens to us but something that happens within us.

That is why we in yoga emphasize reflection and meditation, since that gives us the tools we need in order to elevate ourselves so we can see the bigger picture. And so we can, over time, start to figure out how we can yoke our potential with our capabilities. We can only do that by trying things out, doing it again differently, and then trying yet again. So we need to understand our potential and train our capacity, since life will always involve challenges and will always be a dance of opposites, of highs and lows. If we are better equipped in dealing with the dance of life (in yoga this is called *lila*) we will have a richer, fuller, stress-limited life.

The more we start to look into each polarity of being and try to find a balancing point, the better-equipped we'll be, since we can gather forces from two spheres of being: the right and the left, the upper and the lower, the inner and the outer, the being and the doing, life and death, etc. Then we become humans par excellence. Then we can balance life and reach happiness since we have all we need and we live in harmony with nature and evolve accordingly.

So, yogic philosophy teaches that if we are too much over on one side, we need to add the opposite in small dosages, little by little, until both polarities in us are more in equal balance.

Enhancing Intelligence

In their article "Live Wires," *The Scientist Magazine* writers Mohamed Y. El-Naggar and Steven E. Finkel say that today's information age rests on a basic understanding of how electrons move. That the remarkable success of computers, cell phones, and other devices, such as solar cells, depends on our ability to mediate the flow of electrons through the semiconductors and microchips that control the function of these machines and give them their intelligence. But the importance of electron flow is by no means limited to these man-made systems; electron transfer is also central to energy storage and conversion in living cells. Organisms depend on the flow of electrons for key energy-generating cellular processes. Continuous electron flow is necessary for the formation of the electrochemical gradients that enable the synthesis of adenosine triphosphate (ATP), life's energy currency.

Let's stop and think about this.

You and I have learned so much in life. To walk, run, speak, think, love, and hate; we've learned numbers, letters, words, sentences, nuances, systems, structures, forms, what music is, what movies are like, to read, to write, to converse, to speak for ourselves, what pain is, what pleasure is. To ride a bike and how to drive a car, perhaps. The list of all the things we get to learn in life is so long thanks to how our cells cooperate inside of us. Yet life is something we experience through a lens and that lens is very individual and differently focused in each of us.

According to David Life, co-creator of Jivamukti Yoga, "Every day that we are living, life is revealing its meaning to us. We are taught to work hard to attain goals in life, and sometimes in pursuit of those goals we can fail to experience each passing day as full and complete. We only see the lack of the goal achieved. The meaning of a life can be attached to the achievement of a goal, that when unreached, produces a meaningless life. We don't need to forfeit the goal, but 'all the way to heaven should be heaven.' Otherwise you may be on the wrong road. Life is living life, not putting living off for a while until you achieve a goal."

The creation of the universe is like the growth of a great banyan tree from a tiny seed. No one can see the tree within the seed, but all the necessary ingredients for the tree are there. Just as within this universe there are all eight material elements, these elements are also in everyone's body. Therefore, each body—our body, the tree body, the insect body, etc.—are all universes. These constituents are also within each atom.

Yogic understanding is that life comes from life and our proof is that everything we see is produced by something already living. Just like I came from my mother and father who are living, and they came from their parents who were living. The trees come from living trees, not dead ones.

One of the first retreats I ever participated in as a student was a *sivananda* yoga retreat. During one of the lectures, our Swami started to talk about how modern science needs ancient wisdom in order to move forward in the future.

In one of his talks he said the following:

> Living beings move from one form to another form. The forms already exist. The living being simply transfers himself, just as a man can transfer him- or herself from one apartment to another. One apartment is first class, another is second class, and another is third class. Suppose a person comes from a lower class apartment to a first class apartment. The person is the same, but now, according to his capacity for payment, he is able to occupy a higher class apartment. Real evolution does not mean physical development, but development of consciousness. It is not that the lower class apartment becomes a higher class apartment. Matter is caused by life and matter grows upon life. My body grows upon me, the spirit soul; just like putting on an overcoat. All the buildings we see on the land, the ships that float on the ocean, planes that fly in the air, etc., are created by living people.

Spirituality Meets Science

Many ancient traditions and well-respected spiritual texts are based on wisdom and human experiences gathered over time, and no matter where they come from they all remind us that we are connected, that we are one, that we are part of our world, that we are part of each other, that we are part of the Earth and the changes in the Earth.

Many of us believe this to be true in our hearts and minds and wish for more reasons and facts behind it in order to make a difference, in order to give power to our words. This is where science comes in. Science has reached such a level that it is able to meet spirituality and actually prove much of what spirituality claims. Science can now give us facts and reason for our logical mind to understand how we are connected and how we influence the world.

Scientists like Greg Madden are able to show that our world works as a hologram. He says that if you want to change the whole, change the part. If you wish to change the world, you have to start by changing yourself. The change in the infinitely small can reflect in the infinitely big. This means that personal change can allow others to change.

Dr. Norman Doidge mentions that it was believed until recently that the human brain, which consists of around 100 billion neural cells, could not generate new cells. The old model assumed that each of us was born with a finite number of neural cells and when a cell died, no new cell could grow. This old model of the brain's inability to regenerate new nerve cells is no longer relevant; it has been proven that certain areas in the brain can generate fresh cells, according to Doidge. This new understanding of neural cell generation is an incredible discovery scientifically, but something yogic spirituality has claimed for hundreds of years.

Jeffrey Swartz (MD) adds that another misconception we have had in our Western society was that the brain had an inability to create new neural pathways. It was once believed that the human brain had a relatively small window to develop new pathways in our life span, and after that the pathways became immutable. This old theory thought our ability to generate new pathways dropped off sharply around the age of twenty, and then became permanently fixed around the age of forty. New studies show, through the use of PET and MRI brain scanning technology, that new neural pathways are generated throughout life in addition to new neural cell.

Neuroplasticity

Our minds are capable of incredible functions if we know how to apply neuroplasticity techniques. It can help us to learn languages better, solve problems better, increase the ability to focus, help us regain body function due to a stroke, or recapture some lost brain function from a brain trauma such as an auto accident.

The term neuroplasticity is derived from the root words "neuron" and "plastic." A neuron refers to a nerve cell in the brain. Each individual neural cell is made up of an axon and dendrites and is linked to other neural cells by a small space called the synapses. The word plastic means to mold, sculpt, or modify. Neuroplasticity refers to the potential that the brain has to reorganize by creating new neural pathways to adapt, as it needs.

Dr. Doidge says, "Think of the neurological changes being made in the brain as the brain's way of tuning itself to meet your needs. A simple way to consider how the brain builds new neural pathways as it's challenged by new information and its environment might be to think of the brain as a radio. When dialing the tuning knob on the radio by hand to find something to listen to, you might come across a station that sounds interesting, but has a great deal of static so you can't really understand everything they are saying. To bring the station in clearer you would focus and dial the station in slowly, a digit at a time, to bring it in with as little distortion as possible. You can think of building new neural pathways the same way when learning something new. The more you focus and practice something, the better you become at the new skill that you are learning or obstacle you are trying to overcome. By doing this, new neural connections are created in the brain as synapses that don't usually fire together do so, which help us to sharpen our new skill."

Restorative yoga works like this. We go through the body to shed stress in our bodily tissues by placing the body in different passive poses, moving the spine in all it directions, one

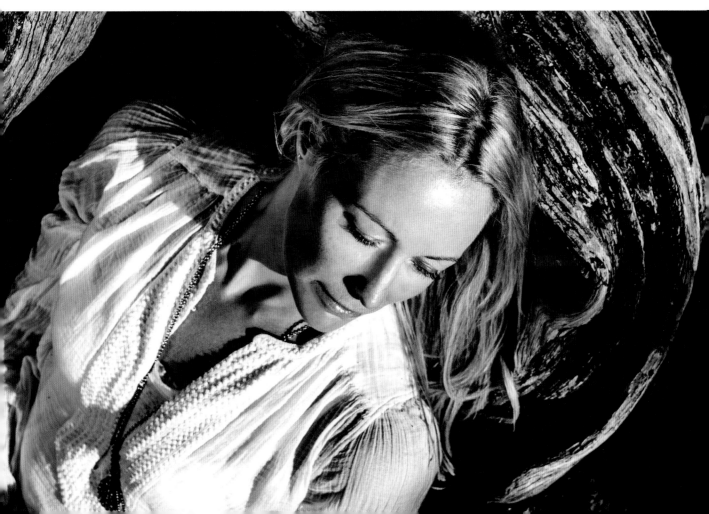

pose at a time, propping oneself up with blankets, pillows, blocks, and bolsters in order to simulate the state where we feel weightless, called the hypnagogic state. In this state, our brain's rhythm is slower, called delta waves.

Mona says, "By completely supporting the body and being still for extended periods, the breath, the mind, and the nervous system begin to calm. When calm, our breath starts to break up into pauses: an inhalation, pause, an exhalation, pause, etc. After a while the pauses become longer than the breaths themselves. Then the mind starts to slow down and after minutes in floating state, the body goes limp since the poses have helped us to dissolve accumulated tension and stress around the joints. That will result in the tissues being less contracted, and will fire off a signal via the nerves through the spinal cord (medulla spinae) to our brain (encephalon) that there is no danger and no need for stress hormones being injected into our being. The brain then responds by reducing stress hormones even more, enhancing hormones of opposite character to lower the contraction in the arteries and veins so the blood can flow faster and more freely. Deep tension embedded in our tissues can start to dissolve and our systems begin to do maintenance in order to function better next time they are called upon. Then the mind quiets and we experience less mind chatter."

The mind can instead be used in a different way. The eyes and ears can be internal vision and hearing, picking up the signals from the vibration of the systems in our bodies working better together. We can then start to see what we can do with what we have; we can start to see what we are. That we are all this, all that. We are intelligence. We are connected.

Life is Code

In 1944, quantum physicist and Nobel Prize winner Erwin Schrödinger's book *What is Life?* came out. A summary of lectures he once gave on the topic, in this book he introduced some of the most important concepts in the history of biology, which continue to frame how science sees life today. One of Schrödinger's key aims was to explain how living things apparently defy the second law of thermodynamics—according to which all order in the universe tends to break down. At a time when it was thought that proteins, not DNA, were the hereditary material, Schrödinger argued the genetic material had to have a non-repetitive molecular structure. He claimed that this structure flowed from the fact that a molecule must contain a unique code-script that determines the entire pattern of the individual's future development and of its functioning in the mature state.

This was the first clear suggestion that genes contained some kind of "code," although Schrödinger's meaning was apparently not exactly the same as ours—he did not suggest there was a correlation between each part of the "code-script" and precise biochemical reactions.

Thanks to Schrödinger, life had become information, and genes were the bearers of that information, carrying it in a tiny, complex code inside every cell of our bodies.

In Tantric philosophy, Karma is why you're here. Karma, or action, is the force that causes us to exist on this plane of existence. Karma is our code. You're here in order to work out the seeds of action you carry within you for this lifetime. To start aligning yourself more with your potential, your genetic code will help you move through life and its challenges more gracefully. Tantra basically claims that the more you can integrate all the systems of your body to work in union with each other, the more your genetic coding comes to life, and you can move into better balance and homeostasis. In the code lies who you are.

Tantric philosophy also argues that Karma is the sorcerer of your entire architecture. So when you are out of alignment with life and filled with stress and tension, you are not aligned with intelligence, only reaction. When you are in reaction mode, you start to believe that life does stuff to you. When you are in better alignment with your life forces and have released the blockages in mind, body, and spirit, you start realizing that life *gives* stuff to you. Things don't happen *to* you— they happen *for* you. Every little piece of your life is there for a reason—to be there as something you can use in some way—to help you to build your life. You are your own builder.

So according to the idea of Karma, it is when we start getting curious about the pieces we have been given, not the ones we don't get or those others have, that we begin to hone our genes and make them come alive, helping us to actually be alive more fully. To work on techniques that help us to be more patient in our search to find just the right pieces we need in order to complete the life we are meant to build.

To get there, it helps if you do yoga or meditate every day, so you can get clear on knowing what to do with the pieces you have. Once you have a steady yoga practice, you will discover what you need in order to find balance.

"When our consciousness is quiet, the waves of thought cease and we see clearly enough to relate back to our spirit. We connect with who we really are."
—Alan Finger

In yoga, we search for a state of being fully present. By fusing the plus with the minus, since that is what yoga means: to yoke, to unify. Presence isn't something that happens once. It is always there. Presence is like a space we all have but sometimes cannot see or use because of the blinding forces of too much stress and tension. To experience being present is like being awake with the ebb and flow of life; in connecting the highs and lows we experience. To stay with it. Being alive to the process of life itself.

DUKHA VS SUKHA

When you stop living in harmony with life and reality it is called dukha. In order to understand dukha, it helps to look at its opposite, sukha, which normally translates as "joy" and "happiness." Even though they are each other's opposites, they have much in common, which is evident even in the way they are spelled. Both words end with kha, which means the "core of a wheel." Duh means "poor" spinning, and su means "good" spinning of the wheel (you can think of du as the root in dull and su as the root in super. The wheel symbolizes life so if we are in dukha we are not in line with reality and therefore life will be very challenging. What yoga means by reality is an everyday kind of balancing act.

Dukha appears when we are imbedded in our own illusions. One example might be when we are too optimistic about one's time-keeping and fill the calendar to the brim with tasks, meetings, and different endeavors. If I make too many promises and have to run around to fulfill them, pushing and stressing, this will get me into dukha. Being in dukha for a long period over time creates chronic stress and tension on all levels in an individual. We need to add more sukha to balance dukha. So how does one do that?

One thing that we can learn through yoga is clarity—*viveka,* or discernment. In order to find *viveka*, we need to balance our opposites in life and add pauses, stretch our breaths, and detach ourselves from the illusions of what we believe is the only way to do things.

So, *dukha* is when energy is constricted by stress and resistance. *Dukha* equates to stress in a human being and *sukha* is when energy is flowing without obstacle or conflict.

"I think this is one of the sad things about life. That everybody is planning ahead trying to make themselves secure, trying to get ahead, be successful, do this, do that, instead of letting IT take over, whatever IT is, and letting IT decide, for I think IT knows better than you know or I know."
—Henry Miller (1891–1980)

MANY OF US ARE AFRAID OF CHANGE

The majority of us realize that everything we have in life will eventually be lost, exchanged, or altered into something else. It is one of the core foundations of life. Everything that exists will pass in due time in order to make space for something new. That's the circle of life. Yoga philosophy teaches us that suffering starts when we go against the circle of life in order to hold on to ideas, things, and people, afraid of letting go. Instead, we hold on to concepts of how things "should" be or the idea of staying young no matter what, needing to have success, fame or money. And when this shifts, then dukha is inevitable.

To realize that everything changes can be a constructive way to bring our everyday problems into perspective and stop taking ourselves so seriously. It can be very scary to see one's own impermanence (anitya), but it can also feel incredibly liberating.

Maybe you can start implementing this into your life so that when you are in an upset situation, you pause, breathe, and remind yourself that you will not look at this the same way in ten years. The bigger step back we take, the clearer it becomes. Let's play with the idea that one lays on the grass looking at the stars. All of a sudden you start to float, up in the sky, and suddenly you find yourself flying in the sky and onwards up in the universe. You pause there and you look around and for whatever reason you see that everything, including your own body, is made up of particles that come from the time they were thrown into space from an exploding supernova. You see that what you are is a part of billions of years of evolution. And that life will continue after we are gone.

As humans we identify ourselves with our stories and roles. This is not only a modern phenomenon. Even 2,500 years ago, humans were trapped in this way of identifying with life; we can read about that in ancient yogic texts. There is therefore no doubt that modern society puts more pressure on people, but it is wrong to believe that there is a new pattern.

As we learned earlier in this book, yogic philosophy focused its sciences on techniques to help us distinguish between what we really are and what we think we are. The path to this discernment, *viveka*, goes through deepening *sukha* and deep self-awareness.

The Different Faces of Stress

Stress is your body's way of responding to any kind of demand and it can be caused by both good and bad experiences. When people feel stressed by something going on around them, their bodies react by releasing chemicals into the blood. These chemicals give people more energy and strength, which can be a good thing if their stress is caused by physical danger. But this can also be a bad thing, if their stress is in response to something emotional and there is no outlet for this extra energy and strength.

Many different things can cause stress, such as a physical threat or fear of something dangerous, or emotional challenges, such as worry over your family or job. Some of the most common types of stress are:

Acute Stress Response—This is "fight or flight" mode and is a common response to any danger for animals and humans. This is what we experience when we fear for our lives or are in a situation where we are likely to get hurt. When our survival is under threat, our bodies naturally respond with a burst of energy so that we will be better able to survive the dangerous situation (fight) or escape it all together (flight). Living with this kind of stress on a daily basis can have a catastrophic effect on our health and well-being.

Inner Stress—This usually arises when we feel we can't change or affect a situation or when we worry about everything, only seeing obstacles in every aspect of life. We can make ourselves stressed, even when there are no tangible stressors in our lives. Inner stress arises in a hectic, hurried lifestyle and after a while it becomes the norm. Maybe we even look for stressful situations.

Outside Stress—This is a response to things around you that cause stress, such as noise, crowding, and pressure from work or family. Or stress from when the environment is not in balance around us, like when we live in areas that are toxic or where the air is of poor quality.

Emotional and Mental Stress—The mental kind of stress builds up over a long time and can take a hard toll on your body. Maybe you don't know how to manage your time well or are working too much or too hard at your job(s), school, or home. Maybe you don't rest enough in between efforts. You may become more emotional because you are exhausted from what you feel are demands, rules, and chores. It can also arise from staying in a bad relationship.

"Stillness, insight, and wisdom arise only when we can settle into being complete in this moment, without having to seek or hold on to or reject anything."
—Jon Kabat-Zinn (2005)

WHEN YOUR SKIN DOESN'T FEEL LIKE HOME

Many people become ill from stress. When you are stressed, the body is locked into high alert readiness, and you feel constantly insecure and anxious. One of the symptoms is to overreact to stimuli. Suddenly people react with violent unrest in situations that they previously did not see as problematic. What is interesting is that almost anyone suffering from stress has problems with accepting it since one's reality is the suffering from stress. The stress has become chronic.

In 1932, the researcher Walter Cannon established that when an organism experiences a shock or perceives a threat, it quickly releases hormones that help it to survive.

"In humans, as in other animals, these hormones (cortisol and adrenalin) help us to run faster and fight harder. They increase heart rate and blood pressure, delivering more oxygen and blood sugar to power important muscles. They increase sweating in an effort to cool these muscles, and help them stay efficient. They divert blood away from the skin to the core of our bodies, reducing blood loss if we are damaged. These hormones focus our attention on the threat, to the exclusion of everything else. Breathing is accelerated to supply more oxygen for conversion to energy. The heart moves into overdrive to supply the body with more oxygen and nutrients. Our immune system is activated, ready to administer to wounds. Attention and sight become acute and highly focused, and our sense of pain is diminished as the body releases analgesic hormones," Cannon explains.

From this point of view, the world becomes a hostile place where we are fully prepared to fight or run. Whichever one we choose, our body will use an immense amount of energy, which in itself prevents the buildup of stress related to this response.

Our inner fight or flight response always resides in us and it is triggered by different events, some less life threatening, like moving to a new house, a separation, demanding children, traffic, a stressful situation at work, fear of not fitting in or of losing one's job, etc.

The more often we are exposed to these types of stressors, the more overactive our fight or flight response becomes until we find ourselves operating at high pitch levels, constantly prepared for battle, perceiving potential threats everywhere. This is why people who are

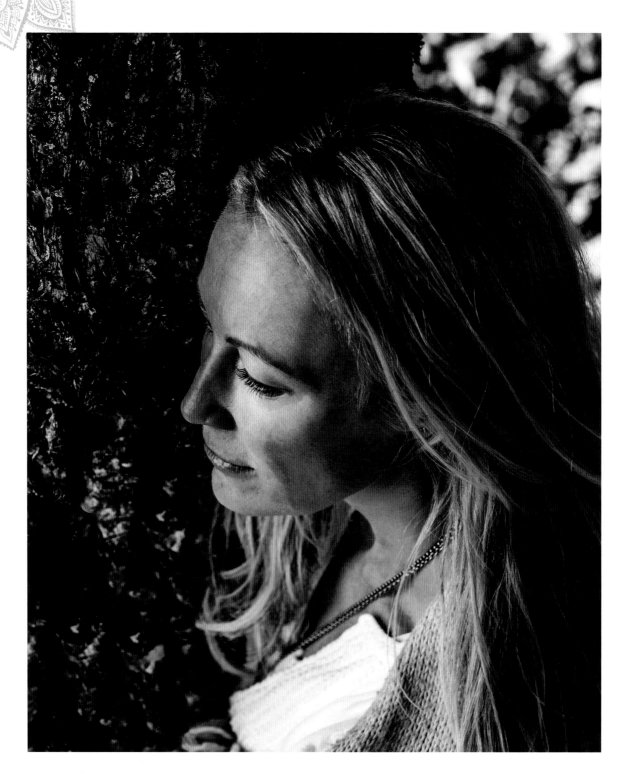

overstressed not only show physiological symptoms, such as high blood pressure, rapid heart rate, or shallow, fast breath; they can seem overly sensitive or aggressive. In our modern world's pace, many of us don't take enough physical exercise to "burn off" the effects of our response. It results in us being left with stress buildup, and even though many of us learn how to control our reactions through polished social behavior, this does not counteract the stress response. And that coping strategy all on its own is a stressor, too.

Life-threatening events are not the only ones to trigger this reaction. We experience it almost any time we come across something unexpected or something that frustrates our goals. When the threat is small, our response is small and we often do not notice it among the many other distractions of a stressful situation.

Many people think that relaxation is very simple. Just recline and close your eyes. Few people understand what relaxation really means. You are tired so you go to bed and sleep and think that is relaxation. Unless you are free from muscular, emotional, and mental tension, you are never relaxed. Despite a sense of wellbeing, most people are full of tension. If we watch them over the course of the day, they scratch their head, bite their nails, walk restlessly, talk impulsively, chain smoke, and touch stiff necks and backs. They lack awareness of their inner tension. Often their sleep is worried and restless and when they wake up they are exhausted. In order to relax completely, the inner tensions of the body, emotions, and mind must be released.

The antidote to stress is relaxation. To relax is to rest. Deeply. This rest is different from sleep. Deep states of sleep involve periods of dreaming that increase muscular tension. Deep relaxation is a state in which there is no movement, no effort, and the brain is quiet.

Conflict in the mind creates stress in the body. Stress invades the soft tissue causing muscles and soft tissue to contract and tighten. When layers of tissue do not slide easily around each other, adhesions form. Tissues become sticky, choking oxygen, creating *dukha*. Restorative yoga gives us the tools to limit the restrictions of flow and learn how to release stress and tension in the body.

STRESS AND THE BRAIN
Claire Gaudry, Director of Brain Brilliance, writes that from the brain's viewpoint, everything can be perceived as stress. From walking down the street to handing a difficult report in on time, it is all a question of the degree of stimulation and the level of threat

perceived during that stimulation. She says, "We all know that our brain is responsible for the control of our physiology, our movements, our thoughts and emotions. In response to what is perceived as a stressful stimulation, the brain triggers the biological reactions necessary to put the individual experiencing stress on alert, engaging the fight or flight response of the sympathetic nervous system (SNS) as well as the biochemical cascade of reactions (driven by the Hypothalamus-Pituitary-Adrenal axis) which leads to the activation of the adrenal gland, the release of circulating cortisol, and the well-known consequences of increased heartbeat, increased blood pressure, etc."

Gaudry says it is important to realize that as the brain is fast reacting in creating the fight or flight response, it is slow to shut down. At normal levels, the cortisol release has an inhibitory feedback effect on the hypothalamus and the pituitary gland of the HPA axis and helps shut the fight or flight response. The problem comes in our current lifestyles with the constant stimulation of the fight or flight response, which keeps our systems constantly on high alert with detrimental effects on our health as a consequence of overactive brain waves. Continuous levels of stress hormones in our blood stream engage us in the downward spiral of chronic stress.

When chronic stress develops, there is an overload of the short term response chemicals and the increased base line of cortisol levels is toxic for the hippocampus, which tends to decrease in size, hindering the quality of memory formation, decreasing the brain's neurogenesis ability, and decreasing our learning ability. The prefrontal cortex is affected; the brain's neuroplastic ability is decreased, resulting in loss of higher executive functions, she continues.

Hillevi Borga, Sweden-based physical therapist, specialized in OMT, tells us that there are other areas of the brain responsible for our emotional reactions. One of these is the amygdala, which tends to increase in size in situations of chronic stress and keep us in fear-based learning. She says that eventually the symptoms of chronic stress will manifest in our bodies and minds and can create different kinds of disease, migraines, and poor stomach health.

It is actually very simple for us to learn to intentionally engage the parasympathetic nervous system, which controls the relaxation response in our body. The relaxation response returns the body's resources toward the digestive system but also the brain balance needed to maintain a healthy brain wave. We have the power to educate our own brain to do so intentionally. Once the over-stimulated fight or flight response returns under control, the true potential of our brain becomes accessible, our learning ability is enhanced, and our executive reasoning functions become strong again.

FULL COMPLETE BREATH

The only autonomic nervous system function that can be directly affected by our conscious mind is the breath. Conscious breathing is a great way to experience deep levels of relaxation and to activate the parasympathetic nervous system. Start here and now. Read this text first and then lay the book down and try to take ten deep, full, complete breaths.

Sit in a comfortable seat. Elevate your seat if you have to in order for your spine to be long and erect. You can sit against a wall if need be. Place pillows or a block underneath the thighs if you have tightness in your hips. Rest your hands on your knees. Roll your shoulders back so you can lift your chest a little. Close your eyes and your mouth. Keep your lips soft and jaw as relaxed as possible. Exhale slowly and empty your lungs. When the inhalation appears, let it evolve until you have reached your fullest expansion. Then pause two seconds and slowly start to exhale, and follow the exhalation until it ebbs out completely. Pause two seconds. Repeat. Do this ten times. When breathing, try to stretch your breaths by making the start of each inhalation and exhalation long and listen to the sound of the breath more and more. Pick up its sound in the middle of your head. Try to really listen; notice the sound of the breath.

After the ten breaths, sit quietly for a moment, sensing the effects of your breath. I bet you will be calmer. It is because you have altered the distribution of energy from the SNS to the PSNS (parasympathetic nervous system). The full complete breath is a great technique to bring into the practice of restorative yoga. It is the breathing method I often recommend my students apply in order to start to release, unwind, and keep their minds occupied with something other than reacting, while their bodies sink deeper into the poses. When the body is calm, the mind quiets and the breath lets go.

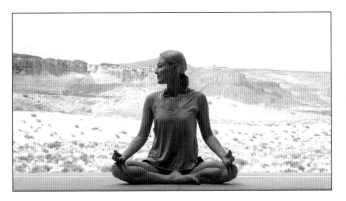

Then the breaths just happen. No technique is needed, and you are in floating state (I will elaborate about this state on p. 38).

BUILDING YOUR BRAIN, BUILDING YOUR REALITY

When talking to my friend Cecilia Duberg, a licensed psychologist, about the brain and its involvement in our reality, she told me that every experience we have, every feeling, thought, sensation, or muscle action is produced by neurons (brain cells). Each time we repeat a particular thought, we strengthen a specific set of neurons. Over time, the brain cells embedded in the process become wired together. This phenomenon is summed up by the phrase "neurons that fire together, wire together," first written by neuropsychologist Donald Hebb in 1945. It is now referred to as Hebb's law. Hebb found that a causality is necessary for cells to participate in learning and plasticity. Cell A has to send a signal before Cell B so Cell A can become the cause of Cell B firing. So every time this happens they start to wire together.

Training of all sorts comes down to this law. Changing behaviors, setting a new mindset, and learning means rewiring your brain. The theory suggests that in order to strengthen your new story, you have to stop telling the old one, and that whatever you focus on eventually becomes your reality. If you are ruminating, a certain trigger is wiring to a specific negative thought. This is one of the reasons why mindfulness is so important. Raising consciousness and becoming aware of what you are doing while you are doing it, helps widen the space between stimulus and response, giving you the opportunity to stay with your chosen behavior.

The beginning of something new is always challenging; there will be a difference between what you want (how your brain is wired) and what you need. But every minute spent strengthening the new story builds its new, stronger pathways. Be patient, practice the new, let go of the old, and you will soon have yourself a new habit.

Cecilia also showed me interesting research that our brain can only process one thought at a time, one feeling at a time. If you practice how to respond to the trigger with, for instance, gratefulness or curiosity, suboptimal states of anxiousness will descend.

Another interesting find in modern research is that we actually get a gift from our ourselves every day; we get ten thousand new brain cells each day, and 1,400 of them are stem cells. These cells are mutants and can become whatever cell the brain wants. So if your focus is on fear, then all those cells will move toward that state and feed that in making that sensation stronger. In order to rewire ourselves from destructive patterning like having constant pain or chronic tension in one or more areas of our being, we need to start setting up some new pathways for the energy to go through and some new roads for our thoughts. To build new thought patterns takes six to eight weeks, the same amount of time it takes to build a muscle.

SILENCING THE MUSCLES

My friend Bengt Ljungquist, PhD in neuroscience from Lund University in Sweden, says there are scientific studies that show that meditation and yoga affect the ANS; the autonomic nervous system (that embodies the SNS and PSNS) in ways that through a daily practice create a relaxation response in the brain that will hand the brain the ability to control its autonomic response. It results in you coming back to relaxation more quickly after being stressed or after an adrenaline rush. This will teach the brain that the negative isn't everything and by doing so, the amygdala (the part in the brain that holds on to all painful memories) will actually shrink in size. It also means that when we live a fearful life, our amygdala will grow bigger.

Bengt also states that our cortex, the outer layer of the vertebrae cerebrum of which is the forebrain, is plastic and moldable. It is very affected by how we stimulate it and studies have shown that with relaxation techniques and meditation, our brain transmits information back and forth much better. Furthermore, science shows that through relaxation responses in the brain, we can lower blood pressure and our muscles can move more independently of one another.

This basically means that restorative yoga (and yin yoga) goes through the addressed local area in a pose in order to induce a central response in the brain so as to stop wiring the old pattern of holding and rather creating a new response, that of relaxation. We can actually silence our muscles (hindering them from contracting from stress and tension) with restorative yoga, in a way that we can control how much tension is being used and we can better control the reflex commands, therefore creating better circulation in the muscles. In fact, restorative yoga has proven very helpful for those suffering from fibromyalgia, which is a sort of oxygen shortage in the musculature. I have two students with this condition and they have gotten much better with the practice of restorative yoga.

Another thing that has been an evident effect of a regular practice of restorative yoga is sleep. Our brain does not have a lymphatic system that can help it transport out metabolic waste that gets imbedded in our artery walls. It's only in deep sleep that these waste products get flushed out. That is why sleep is so important. Restorative yoga can help our minds and bodies to relax better, which is needed in order to fall asleep and get our deep sleep.

Hypnagogic State

I mentioned the hypnagogic state earlier as being the floating state. It is often referred to as the threshold consciousness (commonly called "half-asleep" or "half-awake," or "mind awake, body asleep"), which describes the same mental state of someone who is moving toward sleep or wakefulness, but has not yet completed the transition. Such transitions are usually brief, but can be extended by sleep disturbance or deliberate induction, for example during meditation. This state can also be compared to floating in salt water or being weightless. In restorative yoga, we want to support the hypnagogic state and stay in this state for the entire time we are holding the pose.

Yoga Master Alan Finger, my mentor and one of the founders of the ISHTA yoga lineage, says that it is hard to get into a hypnagogic state (HS) if stressed, and when we feel depleted, it's very easy to just fall fully asleep. To be able to get into HS has been praised by yogic science, since when we are in it there is no *vritti* (mind chatter) and no thoughts (aka, no stimuli on our consciousness), which is a very healing state since it doesn't strain the brain or the body; it helps set up the perfect condition for healing.

Therefore, we don't wish to fall asleep in restorative yoga. We need to apply techniques to lock the mind, and hinder it from floating into dream state, since dreaming is where we activate the *vrittis* again, activating the sense world again. So in ISHTA restorative yoga, we use visualizations (*kriyas*) in order to help pause ourselves and help the relaxation response fire in the brain, yet at the same time stay fully alert. In the beginning of the relaxation response, where we feel the effect of our breath, the *kriya*, and being super comfortable and held in the propped up pose, we come into what in yoga is addressed as the first step in meditation; *pratyahara*, senses withdrawal. After a while there we move into *dharana*; concentration. Then we start to feel free, no longer governed by ego or the mind. In *pratyahara* and *dharana* there are thoughts and ideas coming from various places, but they do not affect you into reaction.

Staying even longer in this state of no *vritti*, we enter what is called *dhyana*; effortless concentration or what is sometimes described as the spirit-freeing state. In this state we lose the sense of time and space and all we can feel is loving kindness and a strong connection with everything. It is hard to explain because the consciousness in *dhyana* can never be adequately explained or expressed. In *dhyana* there is no mind; there is only infinite peace and bliss. There, nature's dance stops, and the knower and the known become one. There, you enjoy a supremely divine, all-pervading, self-amorous ecstasy. You become the object of enjoyment, you become the enjoyer, and you become the enjoyment itself. You arrive in what is often described as the free aspect of *samadhi*; deep meditation. This state is called *nirvikalpa samadhi*.

In *nirvikalpa samadhi* there is infinite bliss. Bliss is a vague word to most people. They hear that there is something called bliss, and some people say that they have experienced it, but most individuals have no firsthand knowledge of it. When you enter into *nirvikalpa samadhi*, however, you not only feel bliss, but actually grow into that bliss.

Another thing you feel in *nirvikalpa samadhi* is power. All the power of all the occultists put together is nothing compared with the power you have in *nirvikalpa samadhi*. But the power that you can take from samadhi to utilize on earth is infinitesimal compared with the entirety. When you can reach this state you get access to all your powers and inner wealth and they link in unison. When you tap into that space inside, you become more and more present in all that you do.

The hypnagogic state has over the course of time and history been talked about and cherished. It allows you to utilize your brain and nervous system better, since it is not dealing with reaction as much. Then you can focus longer, more intensively, and with more width, since you don't have a need for anything other than what is in front of and within you. Many artists, writers, scientists, and inventors—including Beethoven, Richard Wagner, Walter Scott, Salvador Dalí, Thomas Edison, Nikola Tesla, and Isaac Newton—have credited hypnagogic and related states with enhancing their creativity.

My friend and colleague, Hillevi Borga, a physical therapist, sees restorative yoga as a great way to unleash strong-held tension in certain parts of the body and in the mind. She describes the HS as the "loose-packed position," where the joint capsule can let go of the most amount of contracted tension. In HS, the brain gets fewer impulses from the

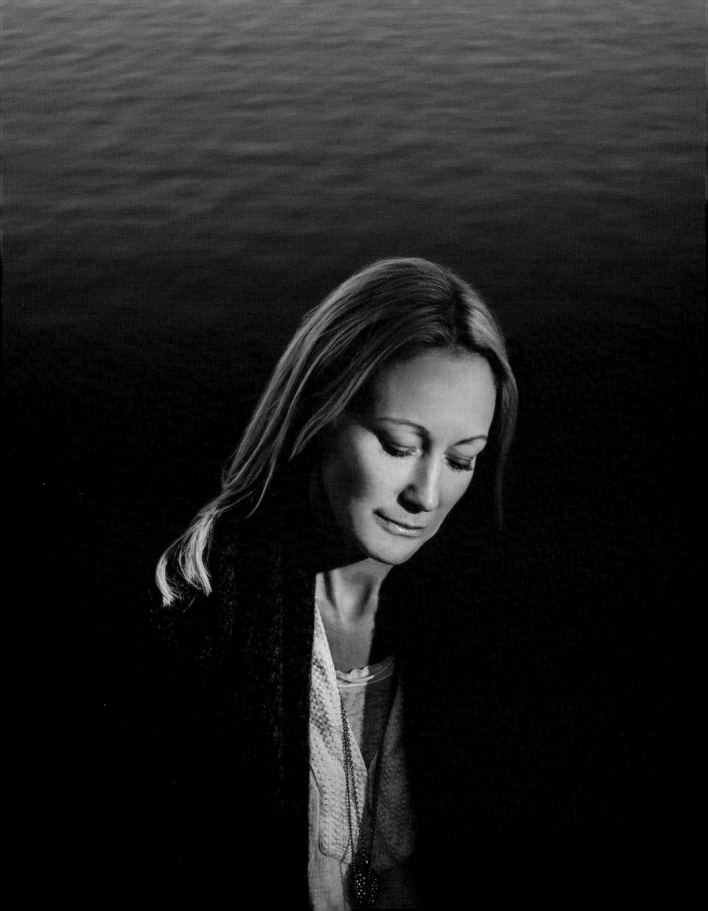

physical body, which is lowering the volume, so to speak. This can relieve pain. However, if you suffer from chronic pain, you need not settle in a restorative pose until the pain goes away. Investigate how to make the pose more comfortable, maybe adding more props or alternating the pose.

As far as pain goes, take it slowly and gently and experiment with the postures until you find one or a couple where you feel no pain. You should not feel any physical struggle, but rather that you are being held. Then stay and breathe for ten to fifteen minutes. If you happen to fall asleep here, it's okay. "You will not break," Hillevi says.

The most important thing in this practice is to start to let go of the contours, the peripheral. It is as if you hang your body on a hanger and let it rest for a while. Stay and let the propped up pose become your safe haven for a while until you can let go.

> "Yoga is a way of moving into stillness
> in order to experience the truth of
> who you are."
> —Erich Schiffmann (1996)

The Relaxation Response

The term "Relaxation Response" was coined by Dr. Herbert Benson, professor, author, cardiologist, and founder of Harvard's Mind/Body Medical Institute. The relaxation response is defined as your personal ability to encourage your body to release chemicals and brain signals that make your muscles and organs slow down and increase blood flow to the brain. It generates a coordinated set of physiological changes, which prepares the body for restorative and long term projects like digestion, reproduction, growth and repair, fighting disease, and learning consolidation. The physiological changes are the opposite of the stress response, and are consistent with parasympathetic nervous system activation. A regular relaxation practice can help to prevent stress-related health problems and reduce physical and mental suffering associated with chronic or acute health problems.

The relaxation response is a helpful way to turn off fight or flight response and bring the body back to pre-stress levels. Dr. Benson describes the relaxation response as a physical state of deep relaxation that engages the other part of our nervous system—the parasympathetic nervous system. Research has shown that regular use of the relaxation response can help any health problem that is caused or exacerbated by chronic stress such as fibromyalgia, gastrointestinal ailments, insomnia, hypertension, anxiety disorders, and others.

There are many methods to elicit the relaxation response including visualization, progressive muscle relaxation, energy healing, acupuncture, massage, breathing techniques, prayer, meditation, tai chi, qi-gong, and yoga, of course. (Particularly the more slow-oriented approaches to yoga, like yin yoga and restorative yoga.)

True relaxation can also be achieved by removing yourself from everyday thought and by choosing a word, sound, phrase, prayer, or by focusing on your breathing. Physiological changes require a good deal of time to express themselves. Repeated practice of relaxation techniques improves effectiveness by reducing novelty, increasing physical and psychological comfort, and creating conditioned relaxation responses in the nervous system. Finally, relaxation is strongly influenced by all other aspects of life—food, exercise, sleep, physical environment, social situation . . . these must be put in order to achieve the most effective relaxation.

Tensegrity

"There is nothing in a caterpillar that tells you it's going to be a butterfly."
—R. Buckminster Fuller

Scientist R. Buckminster Fuller came up with the term "tensegrity" to describe an architectural principle in which parts of a structure are held together, without touching each other, through tension. Applied to biology, the bones are essentially floating inside the muscle structure and work together in unison through tension (muscles) and compression (bones). This is called "biotensegrity," as named by Dr. Stephen Levin.

The practice of tensegrity is based on an optimal use of muscles and bones. It trains the subtler muscles and teaches you how to rely on your bones as support in your *asana.*

We tend to use mostly our bigger, stronger muscles. But deep down in your body, closer to the spine, you have many smaller muscles that, when used, bring lightness and strength to your body. It makes movement come from within, from your core. *Asanas* take less energy and you are more stable because you can rely on these subtle core muscles, not just on the strength of the bigger muscles.

Tensegrity also teaches you the power of your bones and joints. These give you support and stability without effort if your alignment is right. Then we can concentrate on where we need to let go, where we need support in order to feel balanced.

Through tensegrity we have learned that tension is not a negative thing; it is our structure, how we are held together. It is when tension gets accumulated and bundled up in one area that we suffer from it. Then the integrity of tension becomes unbalanced and disturbs the entire homeostasis. We need to even out tension throughout the body in order to feel balanced. Then we feel like we are one body and one muscle instead of fragmented parts. Diving into this feeling in the body results in less extraneous and jerky movements as well as an evenness of tone throughout the body.

The author Steven Barnes takes tensegrity even further into the term "psychotensegrity," which he explains to be the conscious structural integration of the different emotional/psychological aspects of our personalities, such that we not only support our conscious intentions unconsciously, but have access to more of our innate potential.

He sees a relationship between the body, mind, and spirit and believes that in order to attain a good psychotensegrity we need to balance this triad's relationship with each other.

Barnes means that they are connected to one another and their liaisons can be seen and balanced by, for example, reflecting on what goals you have in each category. Maybe you have a mental goal of learning a new language, a physical goal of eating healthier, and a spiritual/emotional goal of being more transparent in relating to your loved ones. You then take action and reflect on how these areas can help each other. For instance:
1. How will being more transparent in my relationships develop my mind?
2. How will eating better help me learn a new language?
3. How will learning a new language be instrumental in being more transparent?

This idea can be brought into this restorative practice since it can help us see that if I bring in relaxation to balance activity with pauses, then I build a better tensegrity in my health.

The Whole Equation

In a world like ours, that is constantly changing, it is so easy to lose oneself. Once lost, we often accumulate more tension, stress, and imbalances. The yoga that is offered in the mainstream channels and social media is often very active and in alignment with our stressed-out minds and souls—a yoga that feeds our sense of doing. The thought that with and through action we can change is very necessary for our survival and evolution, and it's also true. But it is only half of the truth. We also need pauses to slow things down. It is only in the space of a pause where we can evolve and reflect and improve. The tissues in our bodies are designed to do two things: engage and relax. If we align ourselves more with our own architecture as humans, we find homeostasis, balance, and we can live a healthier life. In slowing down, we start to connect to life´s intelligence.

For me, restorative yoga has been a phenomenal practice and aid during challenging times in my life. It's nurturing and healing approach has worked wonders when I, as a writer, have experienced limitations in mind and body after sitting for hours, eating poorly, and skipping exercise. After ten minutes in a restorative pose, I am once again aligned with my creative forces.

I used restorative techniques when I was pregnant in order to breathe better, release tension, and prepare for birth (and to aid breastfeeding), and I practice it when I feel depleted, need comfort, and when I need my own timeouts. Restorative yoga in partnership with meditation and *pranayama* (breathing exercises) and yin yoga, has also turned out to be very beneficial when I need to focus and gather my inner powers before important lectures, long teaching periods, and creative projects. It helps me to go to my inner space and be with nothingness for a moment. It allows me to connect to life and my chamber of power.

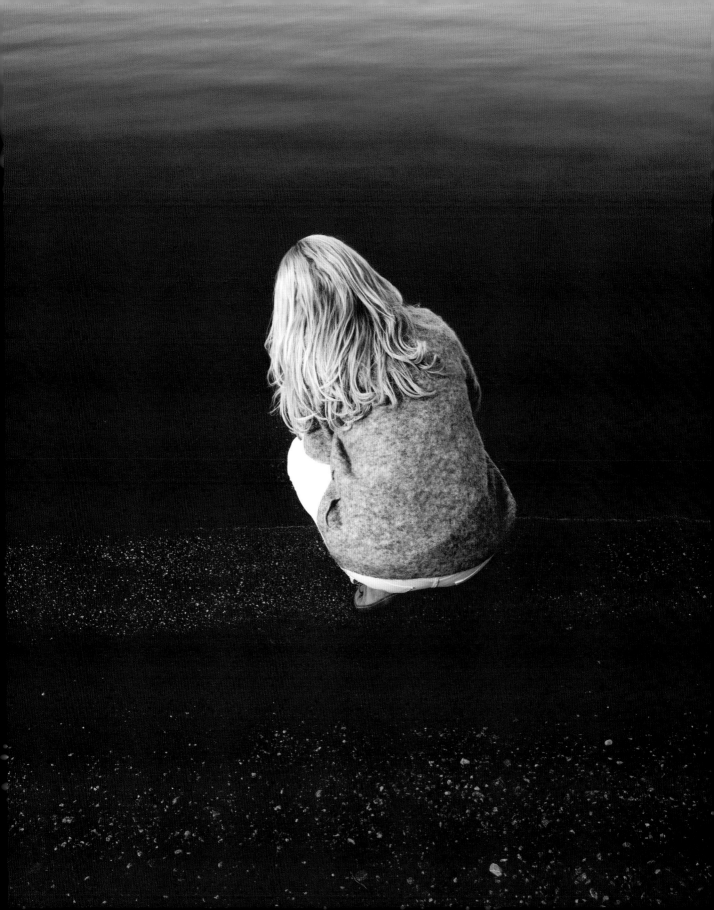

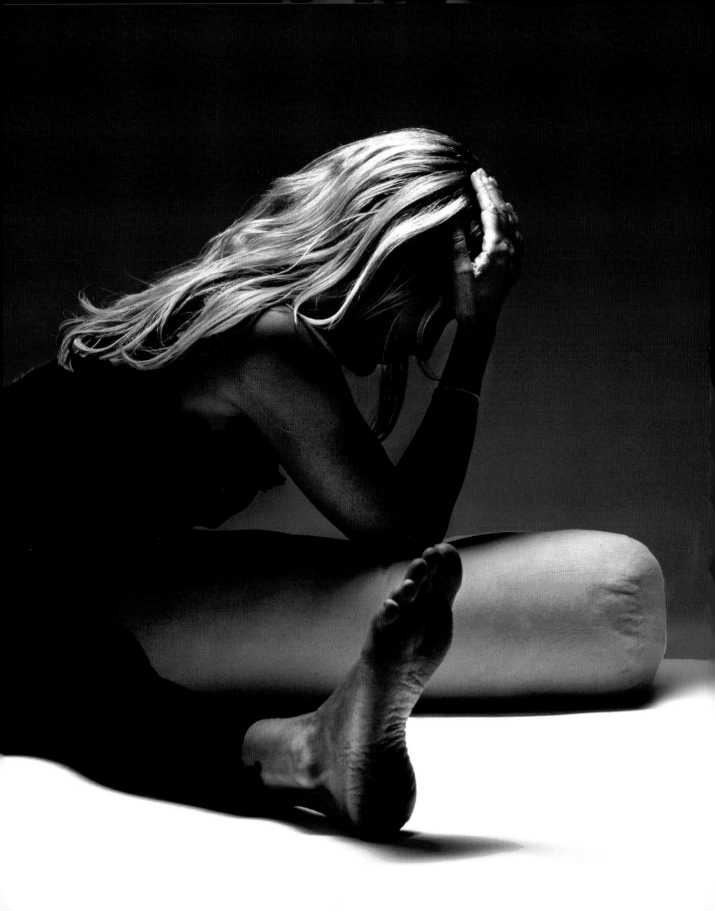

Chapter Three
RESTORATIVE TECHNIQUES

*"You will know (the good from the bad) when you are calm, at peace. Passive.
A Jedi uses the Force for knowledge and defense, never for attack."*
—Yoda

A life can be filled with countless lost moments. As we juggle the demands of family, work, health, and all else, we can easily loose the connection to the present moment and instead worry more about the future. When consumed with what is yet to come—dreams, ambitions, and being busy—it is too easy to miss those things that make you smile. Stop for a moment and appreciate someone's great laugh, the color of the sky, how great the air feels after rain, the beat of your own heart and all that you have in your life.

Often enough we are more attentive to the drama, problems, and what's not perfect (according to your standards), than to the moments when nothing seems to be happening. We welcome happiness, success, love, and positivity with open arms and pursue them heroically. Pain, failure, and sorrow are things we avoid, and we resist anything we think might cause such discomfort.

To constantly avoid life's hard lessons through fixing, controlling, and getting rid of all that disturbs the heart takes a lot of effort, strain, and time from living.

Moments of drama can have value if you approach them with a more mindful approach—they can actually heighten your awareness and awaken you to your experience. A positive experience as well as a negative one can have a great impact on your life and also give your life more value, since you then learn that life can capture and enliven your attention in many ways. In Sweden we have a saying that goes something like, "It is not how you have it, it is how you take it that makes a difference."

The ego gets a sense of identity from the dramas in one's life, so it's only natural that your mind holds on to the pains and pleasures and duties it perceives. And there are so many things that are so ordinary that we barely notice: that the trees grow, birds sing, how someone walks, the color of someone's car. When stressed and occupied with one's own story of life, we fail to see and notice the details that makes a whole, having a more whole life experience.

We often dismiss the ordinary as boring, lacking in richness, intensity, and completeness. When accustomed to externalizing happiness and vitality, you may begin to detect an inner unease or discontent in the midst of any moment that is neither dramatic nor intense.

Finding Delight in Pausing

When practicing yoga, we aim to withdraw our senses, called *Pratyahara* in Sanskrit, through listening to our breath, focusing our gaze, softening our skin, closing our eyes, and engaging the muscles, as well as relaxing them. Doing this repeatedly strengthens our ability to focus over time. We can use our senses in various ways; outwardly and inwardly. Our senses give us the lens through which we see ourselves and the world. And like a camera, we need to clean the lens regularly so the images we take don't lack sharpness. The same thing goes with our human senses. They need rest and rebalance so our take on what we perceive, see, and experience, gives us valuable information on which we base our choices and outlook on life.

Many of us find ourselves using quiet moments as a springboard for the pursuit of some new, more exciting event. But if one can shed one's intensity addiction long enough to experience the ordinary moments in one's life, one will find that they are all doorways to the richness and vitality that live within our own heart. When one starts celebrating the ordinary moments in life, one begins to connect with all that has gone unnoticed in both your inner and outer life. Awareness starts to emerge not only in the more glossy moments but in the more plain ones, too.

According to Mona Anand, restorative yoga provides the perfect antidote to stress because it creates a supported pause. By completely supporting the body and being still for extended periods, the breath, the mind, and the nervous system begin to calm. Different restorative poses can be used for different purposes, though they all help to quiet the nervous system. There are poses that open the breath and lift the spirits when we're feeling depressed, poses that are supportive and nurturing when we're feeling anxious, and poses that target specific parts of the body where tension accumulates.

Regarding the subtle body, Mona says that restorative yoga opens energetic lines in the body because of the amount of time we spend in each pose. We have 72,000 nadis, or energetic pathways, in the body. When teaching restorative, Mona focuses on balancing the energetic centers or chakras that run along shashumna nadi, the central energetic pathway that runs along the spine.

"Each of these chakras governs a different segment of the body so energetic imbalances in these chakras lead to imbalance in our lives and are reflected in the physical body. Restorative poses begin to correct energetic imbalances first by rebalancing the physical body. When combined with specific Kriya techniques they can be very effective in rebalancing the subtle body," she says. Mona has developed a method of integrating the chakras into restorative.

To understand what the subtle body is, think about the inner forces that make your whole system work. We can compare it to when we look at an airplane in the sky. We just see it fly; we don't see all the actions inside of it, or what it takes in order to make that airplane fly, or all the aspects of aerodynamics. The subtle body is like that. It is what connects the internal with the external. In the subtle body lies the integration between our tissues and our nerves, and how they connect with muscles, organs, cells, and molecules. So if one can directly speak with the subtle body, one can affect the whole body. This is yoga's entire thesis. If we reach a balance in our subtle body, our spirit becomes freer. And in yoga, we move through the body in order to balance the subtler entities of our existence.

Restorative poses help relieve the effects of chronic stress in several ways. First, the use of props as described in this book provides a completely supportive environment for total relaxation.

Second, each restorative sequence is designed to move the spine in all directions. These movements illustrate the age-old wisdom of yoga that teaches well-being is enhanced by a healthy spine. Some of the restorative poses are backbends, while others are forward bends. Additional poses gently twist the column both left and right.

Third, a well-sequenced restorative practice also includes an inverted pose, which reverses the effects of gravity. This can be as simple as putting the legs on a bolster or pillow, but the effects are quite dramatic. Because we stand or sit most of the day, blood and lymph fluid accumulate in the lower extremities. By changing the relationship of the legs to gravity, fluids are returned to the upper body and heart function is enhanced.

Psychobiologist and yoga teacher Roger Cole, PhD, consultant to the University of California, San Diego in sleep research and biological rhythms, has done preliminary research on the effects of inverted poses. He found that they dramatically alter hormone levels, thus reducing brain arousal, blood pressure, and fluid retention. He attributes these benefits to a slowing of the heart rate and dilation of the blood vessels in the upper body that comes from reversing the effects of gravity.

Fourth, restorative yoga alternately stimulates and soothes the organs. For example, by closing the abdomen with a forward bend and then opening it with a backbend, the abdominal organs are squeezed, forcing the blood out, and then opened, so that fresh blood returns to soak the organs. With this movement of blood comes the enhanced exchange of oxygen and waste products across the cell membranes.

Finally, yoga teaches that the body is permeated with energy. *Prana*, the activating life force, resides above the diaphragm, moves upward, and controls respiration and heart rate. *Apana*, the grounding energetic life force, resides below the diaphragm, moves

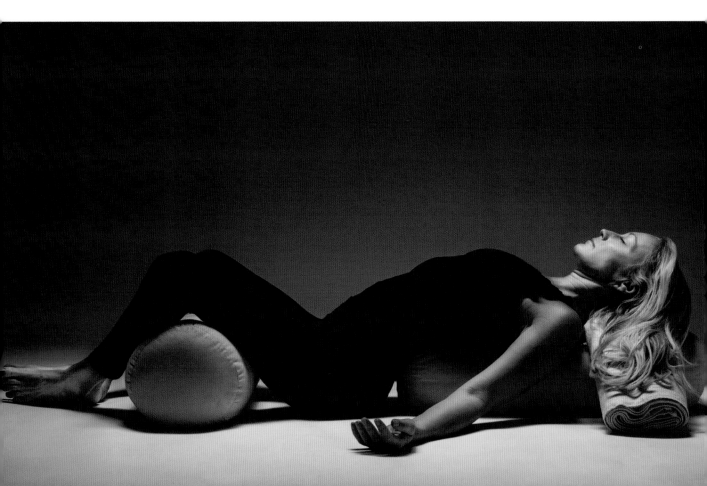

downward, and controls the function of the abdominal organs. Restorative yoga balances these two aspects of energy so that the practitioner is neither overstimulated nor depleted.

Starting Point—Finding the "Yummy" State

In this book, I have chosen some of the poses that I believe set a good foundation for a home practice or, for restorative teachers, may give some inspiration for your own practice or for your classes. I have added some of my personal notes that hopefully will add value for you as you practice these techniques.

In practicing restorative poses, you usually lie down or sit upright, leaning into a chair or a bolster in order to support your limbs and head. Some poses require only a few props, and others require more. It varies from day to day, person to person, moment to moment. For me, sometimes I need a lot of props to feel held in order to relax into the pose, and other times I need fewer.

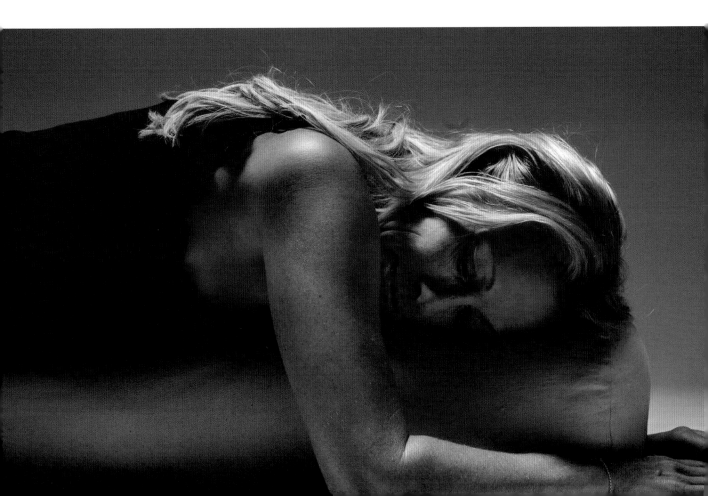

This practice would not be as effective without the props since they help remove the pressure on the joints to improve circulation (via the joints) and fire off the relaxation response in the brain. This practice is all about being rather than doing, yet one first needs to do some detailed propping up in these poses in order to get to, as Mona calls it, the "yummy state."

Being super comfortable in the poses is very important, so I want you to start paying more and more attention to your comfort. Places where we often hold tension are the lower back, abdomen, jaw, neck, and pelvis. So if you are uncomfortable in a pose, gently come out of it and rearrange the props until you reach the "yummy state."

How do you know you are there? Well, if you come into the pose being correctly propped up and almost immediately relax, and if being there brings a smile to your face or an *ahhh* to your lips because you are so comfortable, then you are in the Yummy state.

Props

The guiding principle of restorative yoga is that support creates release. Every pose is a variation on that theme, and the aim of each pose is the same: relaxation. The most obvious feature of a restorative yoga class is the array of props: blankets, bolsters, and blocks support the body to release muscular tension.

Restorative yoga uses a wide range of props to support the body. When the body is fully supported in a pose, students can relax into the shape of the pose without exerting any physical effort to stay there. They can therefore "receive" rather than "do" the pose.

Restorative yoga props serve two basic support roles: they can *prop up* (support the shape of a pose from below), or they can *anchor* (stabilize the shape of a pose, preventing both effort and movement).

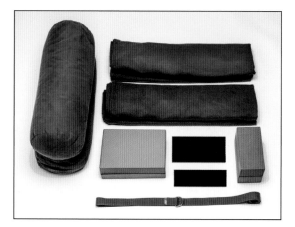

Bolsters, blankets, and blocks can be arranged in many shapes and heights to support from below, as shown in supported bridge pose and reclining bound angle pose. The primary anchoring props are straps and sandbags. For example, straps can support the legs in bridge and bound angle pose, allowing students to let go of the effort to hold the legs in place. Sandbags can be placed on top of the body, as shown in bound angle and in gentle inversion. In both these cases, the weight of the sandbags creates a sense of being held in the pose, much like when a yoga teacher applies a hands-on adjustment in an active yoga class.

I have organized the props by category and the image below shows you the different props we commonly use.

MATS

I prefer to use a sticky yoga mat for restorative yoga, preferably a thicker one for better support, or a sheep's wool yoga mat. In the winter and fall, or when I am low on energy, I use my wool mat, and other times I use my non-slip sticky yoga mat. You can buy yoga mats online or at a well-stocked yoga studio. I prefer to use organic, recyclable yoga mats; they are usually a little more expensive, but they are a good value since they hold up much longer. The sheep's wool yoga mats are amazing and you can order them online. I get mine from sites in Germany or New Zealand; they have the best quality that I've found.

BLANKETS

The most useful props in this practice have to be blankets. You can use them to lie on, to cover yourself with, for padding, and for insulation. They can be any type: afghans, quilts, cotton, or wool. When using blankets to prop your body, you need firm, large-sized blankets. I recommend blankets that are 150 x 230 cm/60 x 90 inches, which give you a great starting point to fold in various ways for many different purposes. The blankets I use at home are organic cotton mixed with wool.

The standard folded blanket is the basic blanket prop configuration. You fold the blanket in half three times until it is about 21 x 28 inches/55 x 70 cm. You can then add different folds in order to support the neck, knees, or head. I suggest you practice folding your blankets as shown below, since the more clean-cut folds will pay off in the practice. A poorly folded blanket will make wrinkles, which will result in discomfort when you lie on it for a number of minutes.

FOLDING BLANKETS:

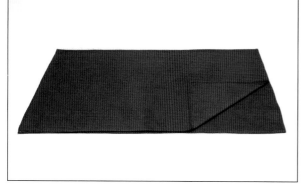
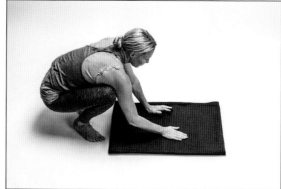

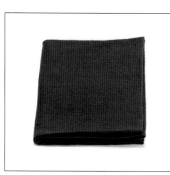

The standard fold.

Fold the blanket three times.

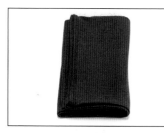

The single fold.

Standard fold; then fold in half lengthwise.

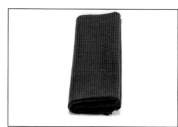

The three-fold.

Standard fold; then fold in toward
the middle from right and then from left.

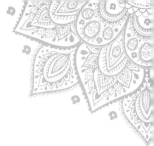

The sausage roll.

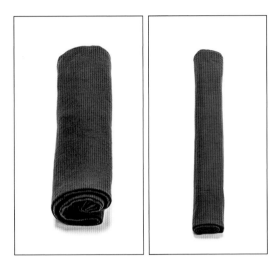

Standard fold; then start at a long folded edge and roll the blanket up.

BOLSTERS

Bolsters are stuffed, round, sausage-shaped pillows. The stuffing in them varies. Some have rice in them, but I don't recommend those since rice can mold. The most common stuffing is buckwheat, which I do recommend because it is more organic and non-synthetic. Since you will be using the fabric against your skin, you want organic cotton or something that breathes.

There are different shapes of bolsters. The most common ones are:

The Rectangular Yoga Bolster.

The wide, flat surface of the Rectangular Yoga Bolster makes it highly stable, and perfect for restorative yoga. Thinner than the Cylindrical Yoga Bolster, it allows for a deeper forward bend or a gentler chest opening.

Long Rectangular Yoga Bolster.

The Long Rectangular Bolster is similar to the rectangular bolster, but longer and not as thick. It was designed to facilitate deeper breathing. The longer length supports the entire spine, from the lower back to the head. The narrow width and slight lift allow the chest to relax and open, increasing lung capacity. Its versatility extends beyond breath work. It is also perfect for any pose where you need a little extra height and support.

The Cylindrical Yoga Bolster.

The Cylindrical Yoga Bolster will provide more support in forward bends and a deeper chest opening than the Rectangular Yoga Bolster. It's also ideal for placing under the knees to lengthen and release the lower back.

At least one large, firm bolster is used in the majority of the poses. When using bolsters, you reduce the number of blankets. One bolster can be replaced by three or more folded blankets. Sometimes a rolled up towel is great to use under one's neck, under the knees, or to support the hands.

BLOCKS

B. K. S. Iyengar's stated ideal size for a yoga block is 9 x 4.5 x 3 inches/23 x12 x 8 cm, but you will find blocks that are both larger and smaller than this. Originally, yoga blocks were made of wood, but now they also come in both foam and cork.

Wooden blocks

Wooden blocks are often made of bamboo, birch, maple, pine, balsa, and poplar. Harder woods will be more durable, while softer woods will be lighter. Wooden blocks are comparatively hard and heavy (they usually weigh between 1.5 to 2.5 pounds/700g to 1.5 kg) but are very sturdy, aesthetically pleasing, and will last forever. The downsides to wooden blocks are that they are expensive, they become slippery with wet hands, they can slide around when placed on a hardwood floor, and they do not always stack very well.

Cork blocks

Cork blocks can be more eco-friendly than wooden ones (depending on how the wood and cork is harvested) and are softer and weigh less than wood blocks (between one and two pounds). They stack and store well, but unfortunately cork absorbs sweat and odors, which may eventually cause them to smell funky and become crumbly or dented as they wear.

Foam blocks

Foam blocks are less expensive than cork and wood, are more lightweight (weighing between 3 and 12 ounces), and are very soft. Because of their low cost, durability, and ease of cleaning they are the most common blocks found in yoga studios. The downside to foam blocks is that foam can get dirty and wear easily, and they are not as eco-friendly as wood or cork. At times, they can also be less stable when used for support.

Most of the time you will only need one yoga block, but there is a good chance that you'd regret not buying two. There are a few advantages of purchasing two blocks at once. First, you will have a matching set and won't need to remember the size, brand, and color later on. Second, you may often find that having a block in each hand or stacked blocks will offer more support, which will lead to a wider range of poses you can attempt during your practice. Even though purchasing two blocks at once will be more expensive, if you need a second block later on you will pay more in shipping costs, so purchasing two at a time can be more economical in the long run.

If you don't have blocks, you can use books or anything else with the same form and firmness. When using books, tie them together with a belt or strap so they don't slide apart and can hold pressure from the body.

In restorative yoga we use blocks underneath a bolster to build ramps or for elevation, but we also use them to relax our hands on, for example in the *savasana* pose.

There are other types of blocks, too, that look like half triangles, called wedges, and they are great if you want to slip something not too high under your feet for elevation of heels or toes, or just to lift a bolster slightly.

In certain poses, one can put the thinner blocks under each hand in order to minimize pressure of the joints in the arms and shoulders. Make sure you rest the hand on the block so the wrist joint doesn't bulk.

YES:
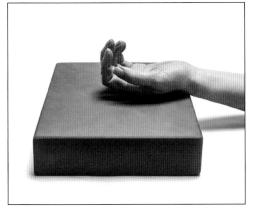

NO:
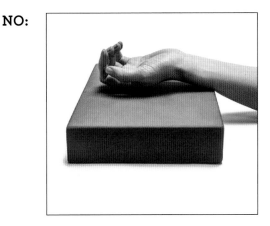

YOGA BELTS AND STRAPS

Yoga straps are amazing. They allow control in a pose that would not be possible otherwise.

The ones specifically designed for yoga are generally 6 feet long, 2 inches wide, and have a D-shaped wide buckle made out of steel. In restorative yoga, we use the straps as hammocks for our legs to hang in so our hip joints can relax, or we use them to hold a leg or a foot so we can release the muscle action in the leg and just let the leg be supported by the belt.

YOGA EYE PILLOWS AND SANDBAGS

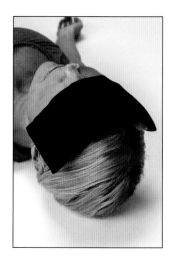

A yoga sandbag is used to apply pressure to the body in a relatively small area. It should be supple and dense and the covering should be strong and non-porous. It should have refined sand in it, but sand should not be too fine or it will leak with use.

Iyengar said that if the head and face are relaxed, the body will relax. So covering the eyes adds depth to the relaxation. Eye pillows/bags are small, rectangular cloth bags and are widely used in the reclined poses to cover the eyes, or as a gentle weight on the forehead, belly, or chest. Sometimes we use them in our hands to help the wrist joint relax more. Eye pillows also have some infused aromas in them like lavender, rose, or eucalyptus. If you like essential oils, there are eye pillows you can get online that allow you to stick a small bag with a tissue infused with essential oil inside the bag so you can get the aroma of your choice.

You can use the eye pillows in various ways for different effects.
1. Use on top of the forehead for more weight on the head; this can give you the sensation of reducing stress in the neck, scalp, and forehead, and can be great for alleviating migraines.
2. Use to cover the eyes, which for many is a great mental stress reliever. The gentle weight creates a soothing sensation in the mind.
3. When placed on the chest, it can help ease anxiety and emotional restlessness. If laid on lower belly, it can aid indigestion, menstrual cramps, and also help to ground oneself.

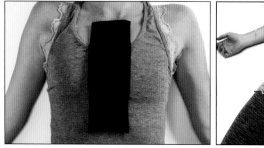

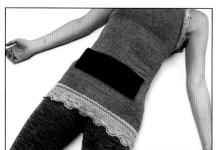

4. In many reclining poses, sliding two eye pillows into each hand helps reduce tension in arms, wrists, elbows, and shoulders.

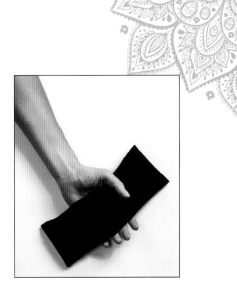

CHAIRS, WALLS, ETC.
A requirement for this practice is that each prop be sturdy enough to support your weight. A chair can be a fantastic prop to lay your legs on in inversions or lean your upper body onto in forward bends. If using a chair, avoid the ones with rollers or casters.

If you rest your legs or body on a door, make sure it is closed so it cannot move. If you have limited space in your home or practice space, then the door of a refrigerator, large piece of furniture, or a bookcase can work. Walls are great support in this practice; we use them a lot. When you do a pose against a wall, make sure you clear the space for your practice and that it is clean.

TIMER
Since this practice is all about letting go and going inside to let time, space, and the external world fade to the outside, in order to surrender into my practice and not be stressed about time (if I have a limited time to devote to my practice), I use a timer. As a mother of two little kids, and with work and other obligations throughout my days, I need to plan my practice. I do a longer restorative practice for an hour one time a week, and at times when I need to calibrate, de-stress, and restore my energies. (I talk about this more in Chapter 5.)

When setting up for the practice, I first estimate how much time I can create to fit my practice in, then I decide which poses or sequence to do, then I set up the props, create a comfy environment (sometimes just lighting a candle gives great ambiance), and prepare myself by starting to breathe more deeply.

I recommend planning 30–40 minutes for this type of practice when first starting out, since it takes some effort and time to familiarize yourself with this practice and its techniques. Then, when you own it more, less time is needed to set things up and get into the mood for restorative yoga.

I prefer to use a timer, either on my phone or a traditional egg timer, though I try to avoid timers that have that *tick-tock* sound. There are a variety of timers on smart phones today, so explore until you find one that resonates with you. I often use an app called "Insight Timer" on my phone. I set it for the time I intend to spend in the pose, plus the additional two minutes to get out of the pose, and maybe another minute to readjust.

Techniques to Enhance the Effect of this Practice

In each position, start with connecting with the Full Complete Breath as described on p. 35.

SA-HUM KRIYA

This *kriya*, or visualization technique, helps you to quiet the mind, realign your spine, and balance the subtle body. In relation to your breathing rhythm in each pose, this *kriya* gets you very still, and brings you to the point where you can start to find the natural pauses and settle into them.

The *sa-hum kriya* directs the energy from the mind into the body. It is a way of inspiring yourself, since you can direct the breath to where you want it to go—to the cells.

1. Practice this technique in the restorative poses after you have gotten comfortable in them and have managed to focus your attention on the Full Complete Breaths.

2. If you can, keep your eyes closed and bring your focus to your breath. Whenever you breathe in, silently visualize and hear the sound "Sa" in the middle of your head and draw this sound down the spine to your tailbone. And whenever you breathe out, visualize the sound "Hum" charging from the base of the spine, sending out the sound to each cell of your body. Very important: do not force the breathing.

3. Repeat this movement. On each inhalation you draw "Sa" down from the mid-brain, and release "Hum" on each exhalation. Try to feel the energy moving from the mid-brain through the spinal column, down to the base of the spine, and from there you send the exhalation out throughout the body.

4. *Sa-hum kriya* will tune your mind into a higher source of personal power that will educate, inspire, and enliven every moment of your living. This *kriya* directs consciousness to the spinal column, the central cord of intelligence and awareness, and

the central channel of energy in the body. The result of this focus is the creation of an alpha rhythm in the brain.

Alpha state is the scientific term for the brain state of relaxed alertness and accelerated learning—the mind is peaceful but aware and perceptive of its surroundings. It is known to be incredibly healing and revitalizing to the mind and body.

5. This focus and repetition brings you deeper and deeper into the center of consciousness, revealing the true nature of who you really are. You'll notice that in time, your breath slowly becomes smoother. Eventually, pauses will appear, moments in between breaths where there's just a pause and no need to breathe. This is the point at which a sense of just floating in pure bliss occurs. This *kriya* is a phenomenal tool in helping our brain and nervous system to reach the relaxation response and helping the body to unwind.

    Once you feel your mind is quiet and the breathing is so slow you don't even think about it, and your body has gone limp, then you can let yourself go in the pose. If you start to feel sleepy, you go back to *sa-hum* again.

    After some time in the practice of restorative yoga, you will feel that a pose has done its work for you and you are finished. This will not be due to restlessness or a feeling that you want to just get out of it, but more like a feeling that something is baked and ready to come out of the oven. You'll feel you need to come upright into a comfortable seated position and keep your focus. At this point, you will bring it to the next level: meditation.

    This *kriya* is part of something we call ISHTA *diksha* in ISHTA yoga. ISHTA *diksha* is a meditation format to help you to come into *samadhi* (a deep meditative state where your brain can mend and reboot without interruption from the mind).

ISHTA *DIKSHA* MEDITATION

Diksha means "initiation," and refers to the physical transference of divine energy directly into the brain, which allows for enlightenment. You become free from the limitations and the conditioning of the mind and are released from unnecessary suffering.

In ISHTA *diksha*, you start with the desire to increase mental focus and circulation and come inside the body. So you will begin with slow-flow *asana*, integrating *sa-hum kriya* to calm the mind and gain inner focus as well as better alignment of the spine. Then you leave the *sa-hum kriya* and bring in *nadi shodana*, alternative nostril breathing, to move deeper into a focused state where you are able to concentrate your attention on the moment. At that point, pause there and try to just breathe (or move through a restorative sequence where you end in a seated position, starting *nadi shodana* breathing until you reach a clear, calm mental focus).

Next step is to bring the energy from the body into the middle of the brain for dissolving into meditation. To help get there, reverse *sa-hum* and instead move "Hum" up the spine as you inhale, and "Sa" down the spine as you exhale. Do this for a couple of breaths until you feel no need to come back down from the middle of the brain. Then you just exhale "Hum" locally, let go of all *kriyas* and breath, and just release. You hear everything but don't react to it. You accept it is there and you become one with all around you. Sit for as long as you can, starting with a couple of minutes. Eventually, you want to sit for eighteen minutes, but as a starting point, do two to three minutes, then build it up as the weeks go by.

After meditation, we need to re-ground our energies in order to activate the body/mind relationship again. Start by bringing your awareness to your breath and listening to it in the middle of your head. Then go to your throat and breathe there for a breath or two, then the chest, navel, lower belly, and pelvis. Massage your legs and feet and place your hands in front of your chest. Say thanks: *Namaste*.

This format is phenomenal and when practiced regularly, it will help you to grow stronger physically, mentally, and spiritually.

The Poses are the Heart of this Practice

Once the search is in progress, something will be found.
—Unknown

All the restorative poses cultivate the ability to be attentive, allowing you to slowly become better at noticing where and how you are holding onto tension. When you have identified this, you can consciously start to release it. The more you are able to release, the more you will discover that a space is created inside from which you make your life choices. Through this practice, you will connect to your body´s natural rhythm and by living in that rhythm you will have the foundation for great health.

The poses shown below are illustrated without a covering blanket, to make the setup visible for you. However, after you have entered the pose, put a blanket on top of yourself to keep warm and also for the additional weight on top of the body, which will help you to release tension and increase the chance for the relaxation response to be evoked.

BASIC RELAXATION POSE: SUPPORTED *SAVASANA*

This pose is the foundation of the restorative poses, since it offers deliberate stillness and solitude. Begin by creating outer stillness: lie down and aim to quiet the movements of the physical body. This will make the entrance to your inner landscape accessible. You will first discover that nothing is still; the heart beats, the belly moves from the breathing, blood moves through the arteries and veins, and the mind jumps from thought to thought. As the props help to receive the contraction in your muscles, tension will start to dissolve, your nervous system receives fewer messages, and you start to become more still and aware of what is happening in the body and mind in each moment.

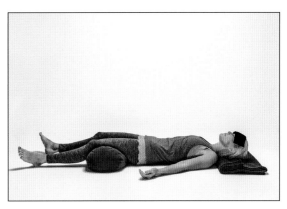

You might think you don't have time for more than five minutes in this pose. But the less time you think you have, the more you need this pose. It is great after a long day's work, after exercise, and when you are exhausted or stressed.

Props:
Standard fold blanket under the neck

Optional props:
1 each: eye bag, sausage roll blanket, extra blanket to cover, timer, bolster

Setting up:
Begin by sitting on your mat and placing a standard fold blanket behind you for your neck and head to rest upon. Then place the sausage rolled blanket or a bolster under your knees/back/thighs, then lie down and make yourself comfortable. Cover yourself with a blanket so it covers your legs, torso, and chest. Focus on the neck; your chin should be slightly lower than your forehead, so make sure the blanket gets placed so you can feel the "yumminess" when your shoulders release and your jaw and face can soften. Place the

eye bag on the forehead, over the eyes, or on the chest or belly. You can have more than one eye pillow, or two or more on the places I just suggested for maximum support. Then move your buttocks underneath the pelvis and shoulder blades underneath the chest. Release your arms to the floor, angled evenly relative to the midline of torso. Turn arms outward and stretch them away from the space between the shoulder blades. Rest the backs of your hands on the floor and allow them to relax. When they do, your fingers will curl.

There are several variations of this pose. You can have a bolster under your knees to get more release in your pelvis, or a rolled up blanket under your knees (the sausage roll), or a standard fold under your head and neck.

Another variation is to cover your body with a blanket like a cocoon. Then put blocks under your hands and place an eye pillow in each hand, and one on top of the eyes. This variation is really yummy on those days when you need to feel held and unwind on a deeper level.

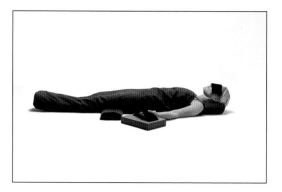

In *savasana* it's essential that the body be placed in a neutral position. Observe your position. Inhale and slowly extend the right leg, then the left, pushing through the heels. Then let them go; melt into the floor. The most important thing is that you feel supported by the props and that they take away all pressure on your body.

In the pose:
In addition to quieting the physical body in *savasana*, it's also necessary to pacify the sense organs. Soften the root of the tongue, the nostrils, the channels of the inner ears, and the skin of the forehead, especially around the bridge of the nose between the eyebrows. Let your eyes sink to the back of your head, then turn them downward to gaze at the heart. Release your brain to the back of the head. Soften your jaw. Swallow. Start integrating the full complete breath and the *sa-hum kriya*. This position will quiet the frontal lobes of the brain. You use the *kriyas* and the breath until the mind settles and the body relaxes. Then you can let them go.

Stay in this pose for a minimum of 5 minutes, up to 30 minutes of practice. I recommend 7–10 minutes minimum if you use this pose in a sequence, and 20–40 minutes as a sole practice.

To exit, first roll gently with an exhalation onto one side, preferably the right. Take 2 or 3 breaths. With another exhalation, press your hands against the floor and lift your torso, dragging your head slowly after. The head should always come up last.

SIDE-LYING RELAXATION POSE

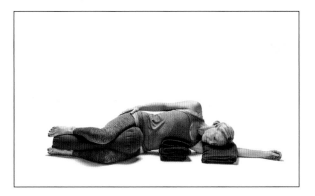 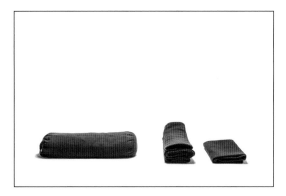

If you are more than three months pregnant, practice the side-lying relaxation pose.

In this pose, you lie on your left side with the knees bent. Place a bolster or a sausage roll blanket in between the legs, one or more single fold blankets under your head, a blanket under your left hand, and a pillow to rest your right hand on. Something that's really nice, restful, and reassuring is to place a bolster behind you to support your spine. Lastly, place a blanket on top of you. Close your eyes, breathe slowly and deeply, and relax your jaw, tongue, and face. Allow yourself to rest completely on the mat and the props. Know you are safe, nurtured, and held.

For those with asthma, raise your chest with an extra blanket under your back and also under your head.

MOUNTAIN BROOK POSE

This pose is constructed like a wave pattern over the bolster, blankets, and blocks, like water streaming over stones in a mountain brook. The mountain brook pose helps to aid and free up breathing, and since it has support under the knees, chest, and neck, the belly, heart, and throat circulation opens.

In this pose, your head is below the heart with the cervical spine in extension, or backbending. When you come into the pose, make sure your head is back so your throat is open like your chest and belly.

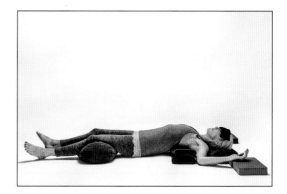

Setting up*:*
Sit on your mat. Place a bolster under your legs, then two single-fold blankets behind you, on top of each other. Then place the sausage roll above the blankets. Lie down and try the placement out. If you feel overarched, just use one single-fold blanket. Scan your body and make sure you are super comfortable. Your neck should be totally supported and the bolster under your legs helps to support the lower back. It is very important that your neck can relax. When in the pose, close your eyes, relax the jaw, chin, and the muscles behind the ears. Allow your mouth and tongue to relax. With each exhalation, allow your belly to drop toward the spine. Imagine your body softening and dissolving, try to let go of all the words in your head, and just enjoy flotation inside yourself.

Practice this pose for 5–15 minutes. If your back is stiff, just start with a couple of minutes and gradually increase holding time when you feel you can.

If you feel discomfort, never just sit up; roll over to one side and then gently sit back up so you don't hurt any discs or vertebrae. To come out of the pose, you gently and slowly roll to one side, pause, and come slowly back to sitting.

Props:
Bolster, two single-fold blankets, long roll blanket (sausage roll), eye bag, blocks, and a blanket to cover.

Benefits:
Helps alleviate fatigue, agitation, and insomnia, aids good posture, and helps to improve better breathing patterns and circulation in the spine and neck.

Contraindications:
Skip this pose if you have a problem with putting your neck in extension, if you have spine injuries, disc disease, are more than three months pregnant, or if you suffer from high anxiety.

SUPPORTED CHILD'S POSE

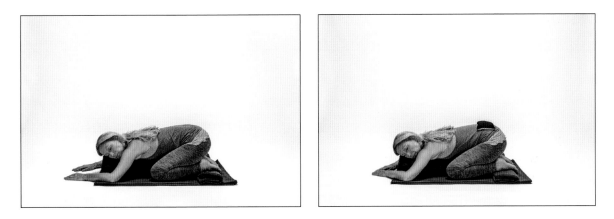

A supported child's pose (*balasana*) is a phenomenal option if your lower back aches from sitting or standing. It is especially effective when sequenced after backbends and twists, which arch the spine. After bending forward or flexing forward, this pose provides great counterbalancing for the spine.

Supported child's pose helps you to release tension in the shoulders and lower back and also quiets the mind and increases the sense of inner security. This pose allows your inner energy to curl up and reconnect with feelings of release and support. Do not skip this pose just because it looks too simple; it is a great pose for releasing lots of tension in lower back, spine, and belly.

Props:
1 bolster, 1–2 blankets, sandbag

Setting up:
Kneel on the mat, touch your big toes together, and sit back on your heels.

Exhale and lay your torso down between your thighs. Broaden your sacrum across the back of your pelvis and narrow your hip points toward the navel, so that they nestle down onto the inner thighs. Lengthen your tailbone away from the back of the pelvis while you lift the base of your skull away from the back of your neck. Rest your head toward one side for half the time of the pose, then alternate to the other side for the other half of the pose. Relax your shoulders, jaw, and belly and ease into the props underneath you. If you feel a strain in the lower back, place another bolster under you so you release more tension in the spine, shoulders, hips, and knees.

This is a great resting pose. Stay anywhere from 5-20 minutes. To come up, first lengthen the front torso, and then with an inhalation, lift from the tailbone as it presses down and into the pelvis.

Gently come back up halfway with the head heavy, then slowly shift back to a sitting position. Move onto all fours and, if the knees are a little sore, come into downward dog pose for a couple of breaths to counterpose.

While in the pose, if you start to sense discomfort in your knees, ankles, or the tops of your feet, then place a sausage roll under the arch of your feet so they hang over the blanket and/or place rolled towels into the bend of your knees to create more space in the knee joint.

Benefits:
Quiets the mind, reduces tension and stress in shoulders and lower back, and relieves bloating and restlessness.

Contraindications:
Severe spinal injuries, disc disease, and unsafe when more than three months pregnant.

UPAVISTHA KONASANA/SUPPORTED SEATED ANGLE POSE
This forward fold, supported, seated angle pose soothes the nervous system, quiets the mind, and increases circulation in legs and pelvis. This pose has been reported to be very effective in relieving headaches and insomnia, and the pressure on the forehead helps enhance relaxation—great after traveling or business.

On a general note, forward folds bring calmness to the elimination and digestion organs such as stomach, liver, and intestines, which are all located in the front of the body. Forward folds counterbalance backbends, which have a more squeezing effect on the spine and liver/kidneys.

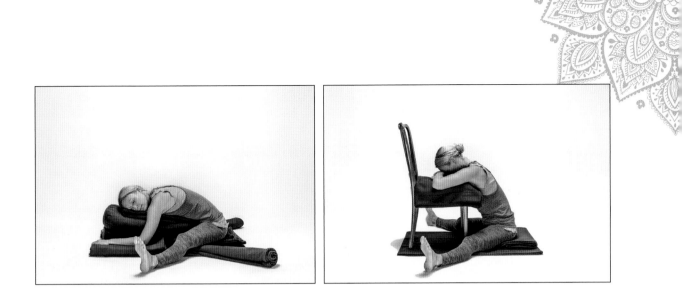

Forward folds open the lower back, which can be beneficial after hours of sitting still or after traveling. This pose is also lovely when one menstruates since it relieves tension in the lower back and pelvis, and if you are pregnant this might be a lovely pose for you to integrate into your practice. Just make sure you have enough room for the belly.

Setting up:
Sit on your mat or the floor (not on a cold floor; if necessary, sit on a pillow or blanket) with legs apart and set up the bolsters between the legs. I like the variation of putting the sausage roll blankets under the knees, which helps to create more relaxation and tension reduction in the legs. Try for yourself and see what it feels like. If it is yummy then yes! Make sure the pelvis is tilted forward. If not, elevate the seat with pillows or blankets. Lean toward the bolsters and if you feel a lot of tightness, then lean on the seat of a chair. If you have pillows or extra blankets, slide them in under your hands and forearms in order to increase the release in the shoulders, thoracic spine, and chest.

Prop your head up so your neck and shoulders don't strain. Either lean the head toward one side for half the time and then change, or lean your forehead on your hands. Make sure you can soften the jaw, face, and shoulders. When you rotate the head from one side to another, do it very slowly and with the head bowing gently.

When you are there, just allow yourself to melt into the seat, into the breath. Use *sa hum* to create an inner environment where you feel you can enter your insides like you enter a sacred temple. Remain there and just allow yourself to soften and leave the outside world behind for a while.

Benefits:
Calms mental agitation, tension in legs/pelvis/back, and relieves headaches and insomnia.

Contraindications:
When you have spinal or disc injuries, or if you feel any sacroiliac pain or discomfort, lower the seat, put supporting blankets under the knees, sit more upright, and prop your head up more. Make sure the neck doesn't sag in this pose, since it can result in neck pain or discomfort afterward. Focus on making this pose comfortable, like you can ease into the chair or bolsters/blankets. You should not feel any stretch. If you feel knee discomfort, bring the legs more toward each other and do not have the legs so wide apart.

Props:
1–2 Bolsters, 4–6 blankets, a chair

Set up for the deluxe variation. Put one more bolster on top of the other two if you need to in order not to feel strain in the legs, neck, or back.

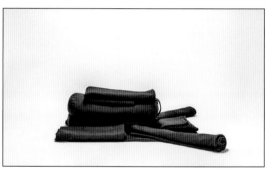

SUPTA VIRASANA
This is a phenomenal pose to enhance the clearer breathing patterns and to relieve sensations of panic, lethargy, anxiety, and lots of tension in the back.

First, check if you can sit in the *virasana*/hero pose, where you sit on your heels. If you feel pain or stiffness, then sit on one or more bolster (in between the legs) until you don't feel any strain in the knees or legs. If the feet and ankles are tight, put the sausage roll fold blanket under the ankles to lift them so the feet can relax. If you don't have a lot of props, set this pose up close to your bed and sit with your back against the bed, a few inches away so you can lean into your bed and perhaps lean your head back on a pillow. Make sure your back can relax and that your head is not tilted backwards.

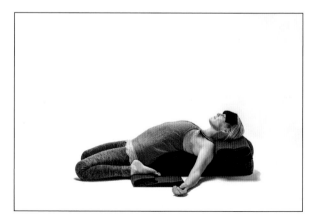

Setting up:

Set up your props as shown in the picture. Sit down in front of the bolster with your back toward the props, and "moonwalk" your way into the edge of the bolster, so your ankles are supported by the blanket underneath.

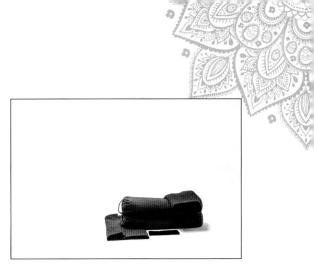

First lean onto your hands, then your forearms and elbows. Once you are on your elbows, place your hands on the back of the pelvis and release your lower back and upper buttocks by spreading the flesh down toward the tailbone. Then, slide the tailbone gently under and take note if you need more space in between the legs or if you have them angled more toward one another. Listen to your lower back—where it relaxes to is the width you go by in terms of amount of width between the legs. (Do not, however, allow the knees to splay apart wider than your hips, as this will cause strain on the hips and lower back.)

Next, slide down your back onto the bolsters with the blanket under the head and neck to support your neck so you can feel the shoulders relax. Use an additional blanket to cover yourself, and place the eye pillow on your prefered place place (forehead, eyes, belly, or heart). If you feel any discomfort, come out of the pose gently and try the more modified version I described initially.

If your front ribs jut up sharply toward the ceiling, it's a sign of tight groins, which pulls your front pelvis toward your knees and causes your belly and lower back to tense. Use your hands to press your front ribs down slightly and lift your pubis toward your navel. This should lengthen your lower back and lower it toward the floor. If it does not, raise yourself onto a higher support. Then lay your arms and hands on the floor, angled about 45 degrees from the sides of your torso, palms up.

To begin, stay in this pose for 5 minutes. Gradually extend your stay to 7 minutes, or up to 10 minutes (if the yumminess disappears, then it is time to get out of the pose gently). Use the full complete breath and *sa-hum kriya* to help settle into the pose. Sometimes, when I feel tension in my chest or shoulders, I stretch my arms a little (moving them somewhat, sensing out a more yummy positioning of them). Another thing that I really love is to place bolsters, pillows, or blankets under my forearms to relieve tension in my shoulders, chest, and neck better.

To come out, first take a long inhalation and exhalation. Then gently press your forearms against the floor and come onto your hands. Lower the chin toward the chest as you start to rise up toward *virasana*. As you come up, lead with your sternum, not your head or chin. I like to do a gentle cat/cow after exiting this pose. And sometimes even a few breaths in *adho mukha svanasana* (downward facing dog) to counterbalance.

Benefits:
Opens the respiratory tree (upper lungs, bronchial tubes, and the throat) and relieves pressure in the head from sinus problems. This pose relieves fatigue in the legs from standing and walking and it helps digestion by lifting the diaphragm off the stomach and liver, increasing the blood flow toward the bowels and colon. Personally, I grant myself time in this pose when I need to connect to myself, and it helped me a lot with lower back sensitivity when I had problems with IBS.

Contraindications:
Do not do this pose if you experience sharp pain in the knees. If you feel more discomfort in the feet, then try to have more cushioning under the feet, or do this pose in bed.

SUPPORTED BRIDGE POSE
This inverted pose offers the experience of something that Iyengar called "The Negative Brain Effect" which, despite its name, is not a bad thing. Rather, it is a cool, slow, and introspective state. This pose is a fantastic antidote for a stressful life in an age that manipulates our brains and nervous systems into being fast, extroverted, and hot.

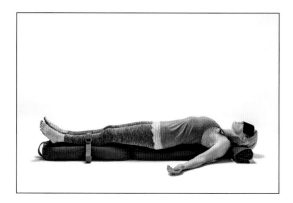

In this pose, the baroreceptors in the neck get stimulated, which engages them to shift blood pressure from higher to more normal levels. This pose also stimulates the vagus nerve, enhancing digestion and reproductive organs. It stretches lungs and, when exhaling in this pose, helps reset breathing into a calmer, deeper breathing pattern.

Props:
2 bolsters, 2–4 blankets, 1 strap, 1 eye pillow

Setting up:
Estimate 5 minutes to prop up this pose; it
takes a while, but the more detailed you are the
yummier the sensation when in the pose.

Place the bolsters end to end with each other
to accommodate the length of your body, or
set the bolsters in a V pattern, as shown on the
variation picture.

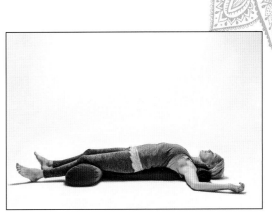
Variation

Straddle the bolsters in the middle, testing the
length against yourself. If you use the strap variation, slide the strap around your legs and
bolsters. This variation is great if you experience tension in legs, pelvis, and lower back. If
you need more length, place pillows or blankets in between the bolsters at the same height
as the bolsters.

If your back is stiff, you can put a single fold blanket under the bolster underneath your
torso and increase the height under your upper back. Make sure the props are even in
height. Place a rolled blanket on top of the head bolster to support the neck. Be careful
not to jam your chin to your chest. To counteract this, make sure you slide the blanket
under your head so it supports C7, the vertebra located at the base of your neck, near the
shoulders.

For days when you feel lethargic, you could try the variation where your arms look like
cactus wings. You place your hands on blocks and make sure that the upper arms, back, and/
or shoulders don't lift up. If it feels yummy, that's great: stay. Breathe and start moving in
to the pose. (Adding a blanket to cover and an eye pillow on a favorable area can make this
pose divine.)

Benefits:
Allows the spine to open while being gently supported. Can help relieve back pain. Anxiety
reducing, opens one up to inner wisdom, relieves water retention.

Contraindications:
Avoid if you have detached retina, glaucoma, severe sinus infections, extreme low blood
pressure, or cervical spine injuries.

GODDESS POSE/*SUPTA BADDHA KONASANA* (RECLINED BOUND ANGLE POSE)

If you don't have time for a long practice, even one pose—ideally a heart-opener—can ease stress and boost *ojas*, vitality. The seat of *ojas* is in the heart center, according to Ayurveda. Try a restorative backbend, such as the reclining bound angle pose, to open and soften your heart. Focus on the breath and the space of the heart, and you'll find that everything calms down.

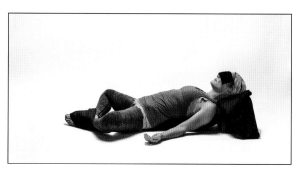

In the text *Yoga Sutras,* the sage Patanjali talks about *Hiranyagarabha,* which means "the great womb of the Universe" in Sanskrit, meaning that the universe is held in a golden womb. It is said that when practicing this pose, we feel a great sensation of being held within this force of nature, within this womb. Therefore this pose is very comforting and one of the most relaxing of the restorative poses.

This pose is one of my personal favorites. It seems if I lie in it for ten minutes or more, my entire being is rejuvenated, and my entire self opens up. I feel it is easy to come into floating state in this pose. Just a couple of minutes of yummy-ness here, and I have surrendered.

This pose helps open tightness in shoulders, helps improve breathing due to a gentle stretch of the diaphragm, helps relieve mild depression, and relaxes the abdominal organs and belly. It is it said to open up blocked feelings and emotions and enhances creativity and sensation.[1]

Don't try to relax; allow the relaxation to happen and come to you. It is very important, like in all of the poses, that there is not pressure anywhere. Don't settle until you are smiling when entering the pose. Then cover yourself with a blanket and put the eye pillow on your favorite area. If your feet often slide apart while in the pose, I recommend placing a sandbag on the feet so your legs can relax better.

---

1. See *Anand Menza Restorative Training Manual*:
Mona Anand, Gina Menza, ISHTA Yoga
New York, New York 2012.

Props:
Several folded blankets, plus a firm pillow, 1
bolster, 1 eye pillow, 2 blocks

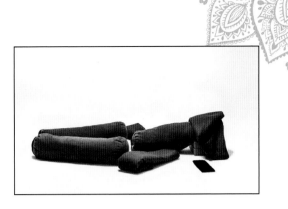

Setting up:
1. Sit at the edge of a firm bolster. Put a pillow or
   block under the end of the bolster to elevate and
   form a ramp where your back will lay. (If you
   have lots of tension in neck, head, or thoracic
   spine, or if pregnant, elevate high). Sit at the edge of the bolster and slide the back of your
   sacrum onto the bolster. Slowly lower yourself to a reclined position with support under your
   entire back. Support your head with an extra folded blanket.
2. Bring the soles of your feet together and let your knees flop open. Support them with
   additional folded blankets or pillows or place a blanket on top of your feet (as shown here) or
   under your thighs to support the legs.
3. Lay arms on the floor, with palms up, or rest the arms on bolsters or single-folded blankets
   like the images below:

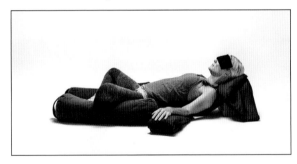 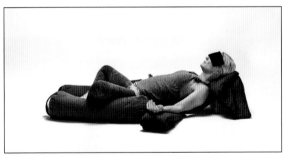

Create small hills with the blankets under your hands. Figure out what feels best, palms
facing either up or down.

If you have two additional bolsters, you can slide them underneath the thighs to reduce
pressure in the hip joints. Then put a blanket under your seat for maximum release.

Add the full complete breath and melt into the pose through *sa-hum kriya* until you reach
the floating state. Then hold for 7–20 minutes.

To come out, start bringing the breath into the belly for a minute, then slowly bring the
knees back together and roll over to one side.

Benefits:

Great stress reducer on all levels.

This pose benefits those with high blood pressure and breathing problems as well as those with menstrual and menopause problems. Many pregnant women love this pose since it relieves tension in the groin and lower back.

Contraindications:

If you have a pinched nerve in the neck or spine, be mindful to support it well. If you feel stiff after coming out of the pose, then don't lay in the pose for so long since stiffness can come from putting too much strain on the ligaments in the pelvis. If you have a knee injury or sensitive knees, use bolsters to support the thighs and calves.

VIPARITA KARANI

This pose is sometimes described as "The Pose" in yoga, since it helps reduce stress on so many levels. It is a great alternative to other inverted poses. Here, in a gentle inversion, the pelvis and torso are supported in a slight backbend while the wall supports the legs. With the help of gravity, the shape of the pose creates a waterfall effect in the circulatory system, as the fluid in the legs floats down and pools in the pelvic floor, then spills over to the chest. What this means is that the blood return enhances and allows for better circulation to the legs when coming out of the pose.

For me, this pose is very beneficial when I need to rest, rejuvenate, and de-stress since it helps with that tremendously. It revives the legs and relieves the back. My entire family, including my children, love this pose and they all use it when feeling stressed, weak, sad, or fatigued.

Setting up:

Place the long side of the bolster parallel to the wall, leaving some space between the wall and the bolster. Place a single blanket on the floor alongside where you will place your back and fold the head of the blanket slightly in order to create a gentle support for your neck. Place 1–3 eye pillows on the floor next to the props (one in each hand and one on the eyes).

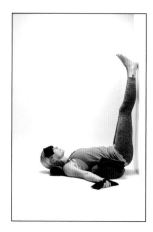

Before performing the pose, determine two things about your support: its height and its distance from the wall. If you're stiffer,

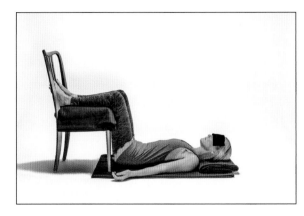 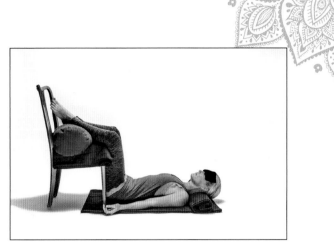

the support should be lower and placed farther from the wall, or rest your shins on the seat of a chair (or even place a firm pillow or bolster under the calves). If you're more flexible, use a higher support that is closer to the wall. Your distance from the wall also depends on your height: if you're shorter move closer to the wall, if taller move farther from the wall. Experiment with the position of your support until you find the placement that works for you.

Start by sitting sideways on the right end of the support, with your right side against the wall (left-handers can substitute "left" for "right" in these instructions). Exhale and, with one smooth movement, swing your legs up onto the wall and your shoulders and head lightly down onto the floor. The first few times you do this, you may ignominiously slide off the support and plop down with your buttocks on the floor. Don't get discouraged. Try lowering the support and/or moving it slightly further off the wall until you gain some facility with this movement, then move back closer to the wall.

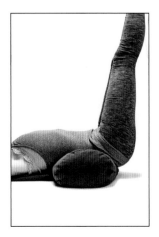 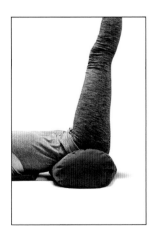

Your sitting bones don't need to be right against the wall, but they should be "dripping" down into the space between the support and the wall, as in the photo on the left, but *not* the one on the right.

Check that the front of your torso gently arches from the pubis to the top of the shoulders. If the front of your torso seems flat, then you've probably slipped a bit off the support. Bend your knees, press your feet into the wall, and lift your pelvis off the support a few inches, tuck the support a little higher up under your pelvis, then lower your pelvis onto the support again.

Lift and release the base of your skull away from the back of your neck and soften your throat. Don't push your chin against your sternum; instead, let your sternum lift toward the chin. Take a small roll (made from a towel, for example) under your neck if the cervical spine feels flat. Open your shoulder blades away from the spine and release your hands and arms out to your sides, palms up.

Keep your legs relatively firm, just enough to hold them vertically in place. You can take your strap and strap your legs together to increase the relaxation in the legs. You can also wrap your legs and body with a blanket to keep warm, or put on warm socks. Release the area where your thighs connect into your hips and allow the weight of your belly to sink deeply into your torso, toward the back of the pelvis. Soften your eyes and turn them down to look into your heart.

Stay in this pose anywhere from five to fifteen minutes, breathing and settling in through *sa-hum kriya*, letting the breath and *kriyas* go when settled and relaxed into the pose. Be sure not to twist off the support when coming out. Instead, slide off the support onto the floor before turning to the side. You can also bend your knees and push your feet against the wall to lift your pelvis off the support. Then slide the support to one side, lower your pelvis to the floor, and turn to the side. Stay on your side for a few breaths, and come up to sitting with an exhalation.

Benefits:
This pose strengthens the parasympathetic nervous system. It releases the systematic effects of stress in the body, mind, and spirit, refreshes the heart and lungs, and calms the mind. It's especially beneficial for those who retain water in their legs due to too much standing, or those with varicose veins.

Contraindications:
Do not practice this pose if it creates pressure in the neck, head, or lower back (if this happens, alternate the positioning). It is not recommended for pregnant women after three

months' time, nor for those with severe spinal injuries or when you have an ear infection. Take *savasana* instead, or side lying pose.

RECLINING ROTATION

Reclining rotation gives us a fantastic chance to untie the physical, mental, and emotional knots we tie into ourselves from living in a fast-paced world. Practice this pose with equal time on both sides, with a little bit of movement (like cat/cow) in between to calibrate. Here, the effect brings the circulatory energy back into and massages the spine and its organs. It stretches the intercostal muscles (the muscles in between the ribs), which will improve breathing as well as create a twist in the solar plexus that presses on the diaphragm, which relieves tension in the solar plexus and thoracic spine area.

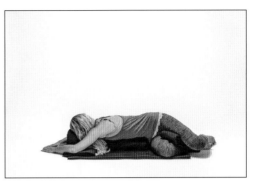

Setting up:

Place a bolster in the middle of a mat. Place one blanket over the top of the bolster and one below the base of the bolster to sit on. Have two blankets next to the setup—one for covering yourself and one to slide in between the thighs to reduce pressure in the hip joint.

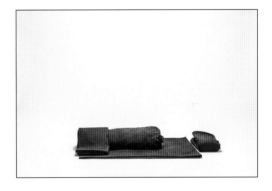

Sit on the mat with your right hip close to the end of the bolster. Bend your knees and slide your feet to the left, so the outside of your right leg rests on the floor. You can separate the legs if that feels more comfortable.

Turn to your right, put your hands on the floor, inhale, and lengthen the spine as much as you can while looking down. Then exhale and start to bend the elbows and rotate the upper body toward the left. Rest your chest on the bolster and lean your head to either side, resting your arms in front of the bolster. Make sure your elbows are in front of your shoulders. If you need it, place blankets under your forearms. Cover yourself with the remaining blanket.

Try to relax between your shoulder blades and use each exhalation as a reminder to release into the twist. Use full complete breath and *sa-hum kriya* to help you to sink into the pose.

Stay between 5 and 10 minutes on each side, and when coming out of the pose, do it very carefully and slowly, leaving your head very heavy, breathing slowly and deeply. After posing both sides, I recommend a gentle cat/cow stretching to calibrate.

Benefits:
Relieves stress in the back muscles, aids digestion, improves breathing, and calms and strengthens the mind.

Contraindications:
Proceed carefully if you have spinal injuries—prop up well and only stay in the position for a short time in the beginning.

Pre and Post Restorative *Asana* Sequence

As an ISHTA yogi, one relies on oneself and what is found in front of one rather than someone else's dictates and rituals. We aim to get in contact with our highest selves through meditation and act according to our intuition and intelligence. Dictates about "shoulds" and "should nots" become superfluous. We choose activities with clarity about their impact on ourselves and others. A yogic practice is aimed to balance our so-called *gunas*, the three different qualities of our collective energy, *sattvas*, *rajas*, and *tamas*. You gain the ability to move toward a more predominantly *sattvic* (harmonious, intelligent) state rather than constantly being at the extremes of *rajas* (excelled energy) or *tamas* (inertia), and the way we move into *sattva gunas* is by balancing our front (*rajas*) and our back (*tamas*). In that way our spine, brain, and nervous system are not over- or under-charged.

Mona integrates pre restorative asana into the practice before the restorative postures. She varies the asana sequence based on what students need to begin to move toward balance.[2] On days when you are *rajasic* (feel restless, stressed, irritated, tense), I suggest you start your practice with getting some of that restlessness out of your system. At those times, it usually feels nicer to move a little before lying down, since just going directly into the restorative poses will be too tough a transition.

On those days, we need to calibrate a little before we start to quiet things down. I recommend doing some flow sequences with deep, flowing breath for 5–10 minutes

---

2. *Anand Menza Restorative Training Manual*:
Mona Anand, Gina Menza, ISHTA Yoga
New York, New York 2012.

(longer is totally fine too). Make sure you work your body, but not so much that you start to sweat heavily. To get some bodily warmth is great, but if your heart rate picks up too much, the restorative poses will not work as well since it will take a lot of energy to unwind the heart rate.

On days when you are *tamasic* (feel exhausted, sad, depleted, sluggish, and lazy), you can start with the long holds, and to finish, do some flowing sequences in order to ground and energize yourself so you can wake up gently and come back to a more *sattvic*, neutral gear.

Sattva is the yogic term for homeostasis, equilibrium, and moving toward existing more in a *sattvic* state in life is the overall intention with yoga and its practice. It is why we do yoga—to come into balance. So our practice should involve adding more of the opposite in a gentle way, and then adding more of it until we reach a better balance between active and passive—*rajas* and *tamas*.

Here is an asana sequence, similar to Mona Anand's pre-restorative asana series, that I recommend you try as a pre- or post-restorative practice:

1. Sit comfortably on a chair or on your mat, preparing your seat with a single fold blanket to elevate your seat. If on the mat, sit in *sukhasana,* a wide cross-legged position, and start to deepen your breath. Close your mouth and just let the breath happen through your nostrils. Move the breath further back in your throat, soften your jaw and face, and start to make the inhalation and exhalation even in length. With each breath, make the breaths longer and longer without forcing it.

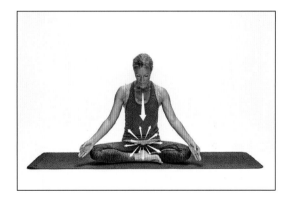

2. Interlace your fingers in front of you and turn your hands to face forward. Inhale and lengthen your spine, exhale and press your hands forward, and lower your head gently. Feel a stretch in between the shoulder blades. Inhale and straighten your spine, lift your head back to neutral, exhale, and stretch forward. Repeat 8 times.

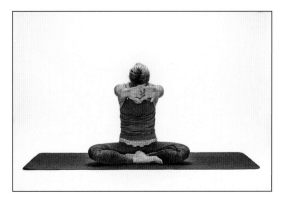

3. Interlace your fingers behind your back and, as you inhale, stretch your arms and gently draw your shoulder blades together, lifting your sternum. Exhale and gently release. Repeat 8 times.

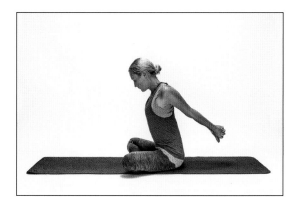

4. Side lean. Stretch your right arm out to the right, fingertips touching the floor. Inhale and raise your left arm up and over the head until you can feel a stretch in the left side of your chest. Straighten your spine and draw your stillness to the floor. Close your eyes and focus on breathing into the left lung and chest. Hold the pose on this side for 6–8 breaths. On the last inhalation, slowly come back to center and repeat the same format on the other side.

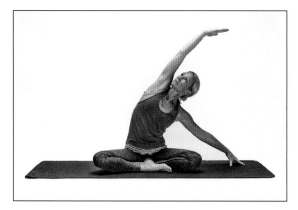

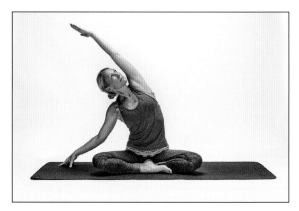

5. Seated rotation. Raise your arms over head as you inhale slow and deep. Exhale and lower the right hand on your left knee, placing your left hand behind you (don´t lean into the hand in the back. Press the fingertips of the right hand into the ground in order to help to lengthen your spine). Pause and hold the pose for a breath. Lengthen the spine. On your next inhalation, lift your sternum and return back to neutral; exhale. Then inhale and raise both arms, exhale, and lower your left hand onto the right knee (same thing with the hand in the back). Stay for one breath, and then on the inhalation, return back slowly to neutral. Repeat 1–3 more times.

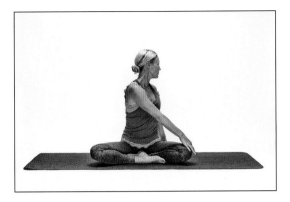

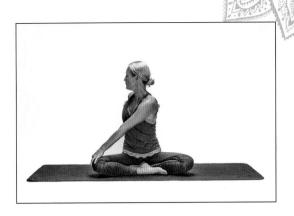

6. *Adho Mukha Svanasana* (Downward facing dog). Come onto all fours. Walk your hands in front of your shoulders and spread your fingers as much as you can, pressing your palms into the mat until you feel your arms engage. Then curl your toes under and press your feet into the mat until you lift your stillness to the skies, pressing away with your hands. Bend your knees if you have to in order to keep your spine as straight as possible. Gaze at your feet. Stay here for 6–8 long deep breaths.

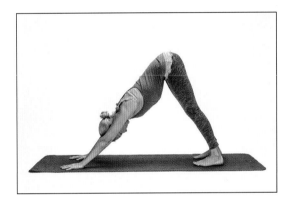

7. Cat/cow. Come down onto all fours. Inhale and arch your back gently so your chest is moving forward, shoulder blades toward each other. Then exhale and round your spine like a cat. Move in between these two poses, keeping it gentle and slow, and close your eyes.

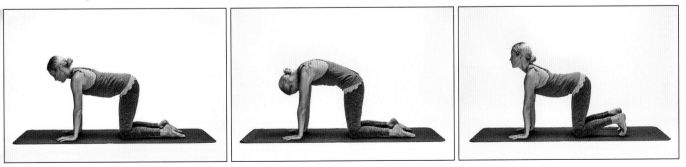

8. Sit in *sukhasana* and gently lower and lift the head slowly and with some awareness. Close your eyes and breathe deeply for 3 minutes (approximately 21 long and deep breaths).

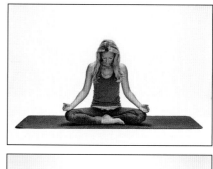

9. End here by placing your hands together and honoring your moment on the mat. *Namaste*, or, if this a pre-restorative sequence, continue with your restorative practice.

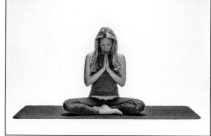

If you do this program before or after the restorative yoga poses (in the next chapter I will recommend how to make different sequences), I hope you will feel less restless and anxious coming into the restorative practice. If you feel very "spacey" and out of it after the practice, this program will help you to move back into balance and ground yourself better.

The ISHTA Yoga Approach to Restorative Yoga

"What differentiates ISHTA from other schools of yoga is the focus on the subtle body and the individualization of the practice. We have brought that approach into restorative at ISHTA integrating visualization, mantra, pranayama, and kriya techniques into the restorative practice," Mona Anand describes the training that she and Gina Menza have developed together.

ULRICA'S RESTORATIVE YOGA FORMULA:
1. *Get supported and comfortable in the poses.*
Use the props in order to feel safe and properly aligned to feel completely held in the poses.

2. *Coming into floating state, hypnagogic state,* able to melt and release.
Use essential oils to help the mind to quiet by creating a relaxation response through the sense of smell. Emphasize slow, deep breathing until settled into the pose.
Stay—Use mantras like *hum* in order to stay in the pose and to relieve mental tension and restlessness. *Sa-hum* helps calm the mind to build better concentration in order to let go and relax into the pose.

3. *Transition to meditation.*

When we succeed at coming deep into the relaxation mode without falling asleep, it feels like the pose has done its deed and we automatically feel like sitting up into meditation. At this point, we come into a comfortable state and move into meditation.

It may very well take just one pose as a pre-meditative *asana*, or we may need 2–3 restorative poses to get the mind quiet and body relaxed enough to start the meditation practice.

4. *Reground to balance back into the living.*

One can feel quite spaced out after a restorative practice. So, after coming out of the practice, come up to all fours and then into some gentle cat/cows and *adho mukha svanasana*. Also, move inside the breath more, with longer, deeper breaths.

When you feel you have gotten back into your body again, sit down and block your left nostril with your right ring finger and take four long breaths, then alternate and block your right nostril with your right thumb and take four long breaths. Release your hand back down in front of you and try to visualize the breath moving evenly through both nostrils. Then open your eyes and slowly take in the room. Stay with long, deep breaths until you feel stable enough to get back into living.

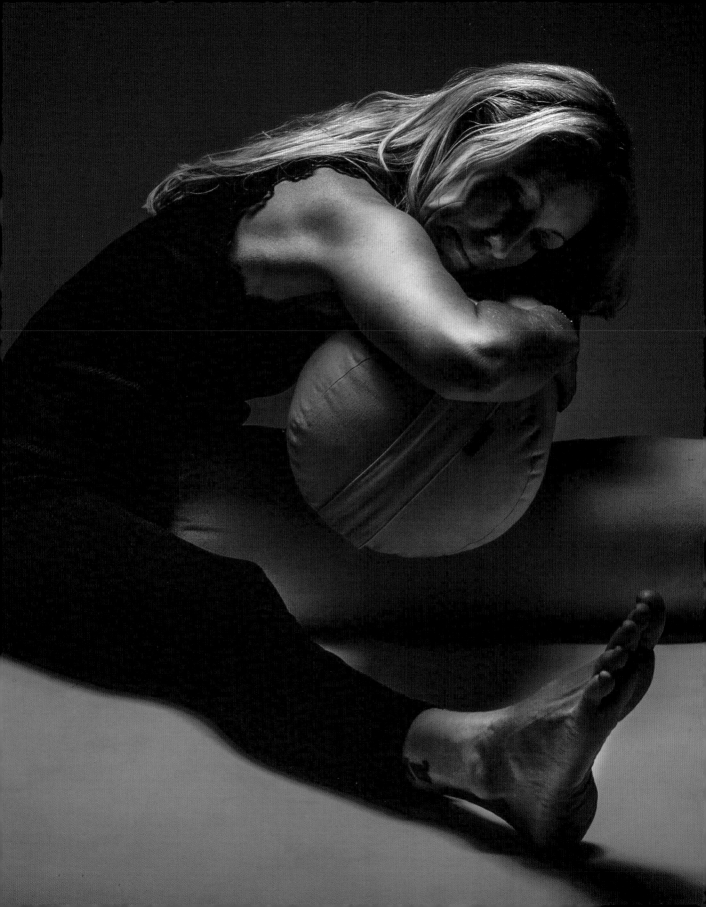

Chapter Four
SURRENDERING INTO BALANCE

Yat te rūpaṃ kalyāṇatamaṃ tat te paśyāmi yo 'sāv [asau puruṣ aḥ] so 'ham asmi
"The light which is thy fairest form, I see it. I am [that] what He is (viz. the person in the sun)."
—Yoga Sutras

Sequencing

Our culture glorifies how productive one can be, how much we can achieve and keep achieving. We act as though nothing is ever enough. This is a truth even within the yoga community itself.

As a teacher, I often witness students striving to go for a bigger, more "advanced" practice, straining themselves physically and mentally to achieve extreme positions, and then ignoring the pain that often comes with such ambitions in yoga.

Restorative yoga is the radical, counter-cultural experience of simply being. Of course, there is the effort required to turn up for the practice and to engage in one's practice, but essentially it is a process of surrendering, an active letting go, and yielding. Which leads us to our first essential point:

YIELDING
To yield is to surrender. Surrender into the moment. Let the now embrace you. Listen to the breath. Be with the given. It is enough. Indeed, yoga may be seen as a practice of revelation: by practicing yoga, we reveal what is obscured by our stress—a lighter, softer, more energized, clearer, and heart-centered Self.

In restorative yoga, we actively and consciously surrender our tension to the force of gravity. We keep relaxing and softening throughout the practice. It is a very rewarding process because for most practitioners letting go of tension brings great relief to our body and mind. Due to this yielding being an active process, it allows us to be in a clear and dynamic relationship with our environment, so that we are very present to this softening of stress and tension, present to what may be revealed from letting go.

BREATHING

As we learn to actively release tension, our breath may naturally become freer, more at ease. It returns back to a more natural flow—a relaxed breathing pattern.

When it comes to breathing, yogic breathing is not merely about inhaling and exhaling. At a more internal level—a cellular level—our body breathes. In fact, it is our cells' need for oxygen and nutrients that ultimately drives our breathing process.

When we start to consciously relax more deeply with the help of the restorative yogic techniques, we allow a fuller respiration at a cellular level. This brings healthier cells which then become more vital. In areas where breathing is restricted, cells struggle to function efficiently, and in areas of chronic tension and contraction, cellular breathing becomes restrained.

INTELLIGENT AND MINDFUL USE OF PROPS

In order to be able to yield and breathe deeply, it helps to set up our restorative postures well so that our focus and attention will not be as distracted by any discomfort. The point in restorative yoga is to remove all discomfort. We need to set up the poses with precision and search for the place where we can relax and sink into the pose. A prop that is moved a few centimeters here or there can make a world of difference.

The way we set up the pose will be determined by where we are coming into the pose from as well as who is doing the pose and what imbalances that person has. Thus we create a practice that is responsive to what is being presented in each moment, always moving us towards greater balance and ease.

We can treat each posture as an inquiry: how do we set up to offer profound support and optimal comfort? With this inquiry approach we remain present, in the moment, self-adjusting along the way. The same posture today may require a slightly different setup from last week.

ULTIMATE COMFORT

Modern day stressful living means that for most of us our sympathetic nervous system is constantly firing without any real opportunity of quieting—we are constantly in a state of flight or fight. Restorative yoga is a perfect antidote. With its emphasis on deliberately slowing down and optimal comfort and ease, the practice activates the parasympathetic nervous system responsible for resting and digesting, restoring easy breathing, lowering blood pressure and heart rates, relaxing tension, and bringing greater balance. Restorative yoga's profound effect on the autonomic nervous system is a crucial element to its power.

In support of our joints, no joint should be left hanging in space. Always support all joints so we allow our nervous system to calm down.

For example, the weight of the bones pulls the arm away and out from the shoulder socket. There follows a response from the nervous system and surrounding body tissues that creates stress and tension around the joint to "hold on," and this is the opposite experience from we are looking for.

When every joint is beautifully supported, the body receives this as a message of kindness and responds, ahhh . . . I am safe to soften, safe to relax.

In this way, our yoga practice becomes an engaging and responsive dialogue between body and mind. I have witnessed again and again the effectiveness of this approach, not only on the physical and energetic levels, but also on our emotional, mental, and spiritual well-being.

The aim of restorative yoga is to induce rest and ease. Yes, the postures may gently open us to encourage greater energy flow, but this can best be achieved by sending a message of comfort, safety, and cohesion to the body.

BALANCED SEQUENCING

Judith Lasater suggests that any well-sequenced restorative practice should include at least one inversion to help counter the effects of gravity.

Essentially, sequencing postures comes down to practicing safely, creatively, and responsively.

Optimal ease means we can sustain the practice for longer. The benefits gained from restorative postures are enhanced with time spent in the postures, so spending twenty-five minutes in a comfortable pose will be more beneficial than five minutes in the same posture, which is set up to give stronger sensations.

Following are some different sequences I like and can recommend:
CP: = Counterpose
(NOTE: always add about 10–15 minutes to the sequence to allow for getting in and out of the poses and also for propping up accordingly)

30-minute Sequence
One of my favorite sequences. Great after work flow.

Viparita Karani (with legs on chair)	6 min
Reclining twist	4 min each side
Supported Child´s pose	5 min
Supported Bridge pose	5 min
Basic Relaxation pose	7 min
(CP: Cat/cow)	1 min

20-minute Sequence
(Each pose can be extended to 20 minutes and be a single pose on its own)
Great to focus your energy before or after a test, presentation, lecture, class, etc.

Basic Relaxation pose	6 min
Supported Seated Angle pose	6 min
Supta Virasana	6 min
(CP: *Adho Mukha Svanasana*)	1 min

45-minute Sequence

This is a sequence that I have benefited from tremendously on occasions where I felt negative, irritated, introverted, and self-judging.

Mountain Brook pose	10 min
Supported Bridge pose	10 min
Supta Baddha Konasana	15 min
Supported Child's pose	7 min
(CP: *Adho Mukha Svanasana*)	3 min

60-minute Sequence

This is a sequence I love to follow on days where I need to just be quite gentle with myself.

Supported Child's pose	10 min
Forward twist, right side	10 min
Forward twist, left side	10 min
Supta Virasana	10 min
Supta Baddha Konasana	10 min
Savasana	10 min

Bliss Sequence (75-minute)

The perfect sequence when life is too much and when you are working hard.

Supta Baddha Konasana	15 min
Upavistha Konasana	10 min
Supta Virasana	15 min
Reclining Rotation, right side	10 min
Reclining Rotation, left side	10 min
Mountain Brook pose	10 min

Sweet Surrender Sequence (60-minute)

This is a great sequence after traveling.

Viparita Karani (legs up the wall)	10 min
Supported Bridge	10 min
Half pigeon, right side	10 min
Half Pigeon, left side	10 min
Savasana on the right side	10 min
Savasana on the left side	10 min

Basic Sequence (for any day)[3]

Viparita Karani	10–20 min
Supta Baddha Konasana	10–20 min
Forward twist	10 min
Savasana	10–20 min

Asthma Sequence (Mona Anand's favorite)

Pre-restorative *asana*
(neck rolls, side stretching, seated twists, cat-cow, downward dog for 10 minutes)

Supta Baddha Konasana	15 min
Supported Child´s pose	15 min
Restorative Bridge	15 min
Right-Sided *Savasana*	15 min

Sequence for an Achy Back (Gina Menza's recommended sequence)

Lounging *Viparita Karani* — 10 min
(with legs on a chair)

Supta Baddha Konasana — 10–15 min
(with bolster under the thighs, and build the bolster behind the back so you are almost sitting upright)

Supported Child's pose — 10–15 min

Savasana — 20 min
(with two bolsters under the calves, leaving legs high. Blanket under the neck.)

SMOOTH AND NATURAL

In order to set up a sustainable practice, we can aim to transition ourselves smoothly in between poses and not to rush out of any pose. When I practice on my own in my home, I use the timer app on my phone. I like it since I can set it for 10 minutes or however long I intend to stay in the pose and then do my work in the pose, not worrying about time. Then when the bell goes off, I start to bring the breath to the belly and lower back to ground myself again, telling my body that is is time to slowly come out of the pose. Then I move gently and very slowly from where I am to a comfortable seated pose. And there I sit still

---

3. The three sequences on this page are from *Anand Menza Restorative Training Manual*:
Mona Anand, Gina Menza, ISHTA Yoga
New York, New York 2012.

with my eyes closed for a moment, just sensing the effects of the pose. It is key to connect back to the body and delight in the sensations of it all.

Yoga is a tradition that spans thousands of years and we have the blessed opportunity to drink deeply of its offerings. Yoga teaches us that we should yoke the being and doing, It is in yoking any polarities that we can reach more balance in any field, relationship, or endeavor. When yoking, we force ourselves to see things from more perspectives than one, which makes it easier to stay balanced and avoid overreactions or overstressing.

In restorative yoga, we may counter the cultural tendency to push and stress and never slow down by leaning our practice toward neutrality. We may cultivate an attitude of real contentment with less sensation and instead encourage a healthy curiosity toward more neutral sensation. With quieter sensations, we may be drawn into an inner space and explore our internal landscape.

A regular, dedicated yoga practice, containing meditation and relaxation amongst its ingredients, draws us into a subtler experience—a beautiful inner journey toward our True Nature.

AIMING FOR TRUE NATURE
The original purpose of the yoga practice—to return us to a self-realization of our innate True Nature, or original wholeness, completeness, and, goodness—sometimes seems to get lost in modern yoga.

Since restorative yoga emphasizes rest, the practice gives us the opportunity to move into ourselves, where we can more easily find stillness and calm.

In the quietness of a restorative practice we can relax the senses so they may be more in balance with how we interact and receive the environment around us. We can learn to focus our attention and sustain that focus throughout the practice, and finally arrive simply and perfectly in the moment. It becomes a graceful relaxation back into our True Nature..

Essential Oils

For centuries, scented oils and incense have been used by many spiritual traditions, including yoga, to set an elevated tone for devotional practice or meditation.

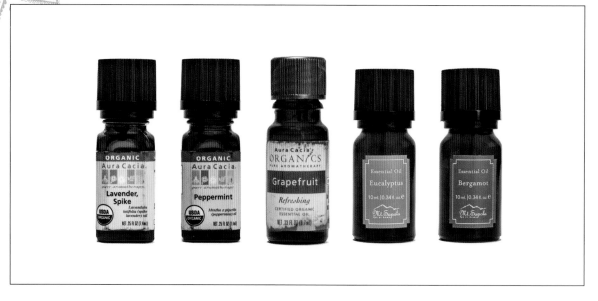

Essential oils are extracted from plants using a variety of methods, usually with distillation or expression. An essential oil has the "essential" aromatic and chemical properties of that plant.

Essential oils are made up of minute molecules that are very easily absorbed. Each oil has a unique chemical composition that all affect our nervous system in different ways . For example, lavender essential oil has 40 percent linalyl acetate, which is an ester. Studies have shown linalyl acetate to be anti-inflammatory, sedative, anti-bacterial, and anti-viral. So it would make sense to take advantage of these properties by using lavender essential oils for occasional sleeplessness and seasonal or environmental threats.

Aroma. When you smell an essential oil, receptor cells in your chemosensory organs receive the aroma and send signals to the limbic system of the brain, which is the center of memory and emotion. It also is connected to areas of the brain that control blood pressure, heart rate, breathing, hormone balance, and more. Experts say aromatherapy works because your sense of smell connects directly to the limbic system of your brain, which controls emotion.

Absorption. When essential oils are absorbed through the skin or lungs, they enter fluids and are distributed throughout the body, where their chemical constituents can interact with other bodily systems.

Essential oils support, maintain, or improve health, wellness, or structures and functions of the body like the brain, the heart, the liver, muscles and joints, the respiratory system, cognitive function, etc.

I use essential oils in my daily life. When something aches, when I need uplifting, calming down, balancing, grounding—for all different types of moods, there is an oil that can help me back into better balance. They help me balance myself so I can stay on my path as a yogi, mother, and writer, in better harmony with myself and my tasks at hand each day.

Try adding a drop or two to a room diffuser, to an ounce of massage oil, or to a tissue tucked beneath the corner of your yoga mat. Then inhale deeply and begin your practice, fully engaged in body, mind, and spirit.

Essential oils can work as enhancers of a certain effect when it comes to restorative yoga (and yin yoga) since the senses are affected in a particular way by these scents. Different scents have different effects and also, since these are natural fragrances, not chemical, then the body will respond to them as natural essences.

DIFFERENT OILS TO BE USED IN RESTORATIVE YOGA

Gina Menza uses the following essential oils to embellish her restorative poses.[4] You can use the oils on certain designated areas like the temples, neck (just underneath the earlobes), under the soles of the feet, and on the inside on the wrists and ankles. Just place 3–4 drops on the insides of the wrists and then rub the wrist to the other areas.

In order to know what oils you need, smell them, and the one that appeals the most to you is the one you need. I got that piece of advice from a teacher that I took a course on essential oils with, and she said that the spirit takes what it needs, since the sense of smell is hard to trick into doing what you want it to do. This is because our sense of smell is very closely linked to our survival, and if we had to think too much on, for example, whether food smells sour or not, we would die too easily. One can use many different essential oils in this type of practice, yet I list the most common ones and also the ones that were recommended to me by my friend Gina Menza.

---

4. See *Anand Menza Restorative Training*.

Peppermint

Like most other essential oils, peppermint is able to provide relief from stress, depression, and mental exhaustion due to its refreshing nature. It is also effective against anxiety and restlessness. Furthermore, it stimulates mental activity, clears the mind, and increases focus on cognitive tasks. Peppermint oil helps to uplift and energize and also is great if one feels sluggish or inverted.

Peppermint oil is a good home remedy for nausea and headaches. To quickly alleviate the pain of a headache, simply apply peppermint oil in a diluted form directly on the forehead. Inhaling peppermint oil can eliminate the effects of nausea and motion sickness, simply because of its relaxing and soothing effects. Its cooling and anti-inflammatory properties are part of the reason why it is so successful at relieving headache symptoms. Menthol, which is abundantly present in peppermint oil, helps to clear the respiratory tract. It is also an effective expectorant and therefore provides instantaneous, though temporary, relief for numerous respiratory problems including nasal congestion, sinusitis, asthma, bronchitis, cold, and cough.

The stimulating effects of peppermint oil have been shown to increase blood circulation. Studies have shown that as soon as the essential oil vapor touches the end of the olfactory nerve endings, there is an almost instant increase in pulse rate and blood circulation. The stimulating effect of increased blood circulation helps to oxygenate the body's organs and increase metabolism, as well as oxygenate the brain.

There are some risks in using too much peppermint oil, including allergic reaction, heartburn, and headaches. Basically, the same rules apply to using peppermint oil as to any other alternative supplement or dietary change: speak to a doctor, and if you don't consult a professional, start with small topical doses or skin patch tests to see how it affects your system. Don't place any oil close to your eyes as they will burn.

Lavender Essential Oil

Lavender is the most used essential oil of the lot in yoga today. Lavender essential oil has been used for many different purposes for over 2,500 years. The Egyptians used it for mummification and as a perfume. The Romans used it for bathing, cooking, and for scenting the air. Some believe spikenard was made from lavender essential oil and, quite possibly the most famous usage of all, Mary used it to anoint Jesus with her hair.

Traditionally, lavender has been used to treat neurological issues like migraines, stress, anxiety, and depression, and an evidence-based study was published by the *International Journal of Psychiatry in Clinical Practice*. The study found that supplementing 80 mg capsules of lavender essential oil alleviates anxiety, sleep disturbance, and depression. Another study proving that lavender aromatherapy improves mood was done on people suffering from post-traumatic stress disorder (PTSD). The results revealed that just 80 mg of lavender oil per day helped decrease depression by 32.7 percent and dramatically decreased sleep disturbances, moodiness, and overall health status in 47 people suffering from PTSD.

Lavender essential oil helps to better sleeping, which has made it a common recommendation for an alternative treatment of insomnia, and its calming scent makes it an excellent tonic for the nerves and anxiety issues. Therefore, it can also be helpful in treating migraines, headaches, depression, and emotional stress. The refreshing aroma removes nervous exhaustion and restlessness while also increasing mental activity.

If your skin breaks out when massaging it in on your skin or if you experience trouble breathing, then shower it off and avoid this oil. You can try other oils like Sandalwood or Bergamot.

Grapefruit
Like the fruit itself, the essential oil of grapefruit is rich in antioxidants. Primarily, it has a wealth of Vitamin C. This vitamin, combined with the other antioxidant components present in grapefruit essential oil, boosts our immune system and fights against the activity of free radicals. This oil is effective in protecting the body from all harm done by various oxidants and toxins, including premature aging, degeneration of tissues, macular degeneration, loss of vision and hearing, mental and physical sluggishness, nervous disorders, and other related problems.

This oil stimulates the body in a variety of ways. It has stimulating effects on both the body and the mind. It stimulates the brain by making it active and gives new direction to thoughts as well as stimulates endocrinal glands and promotes proper secretion of hormones and enzymes, thereby keeping your body's entire metabolism in proper order. It also stimulates the nervous system and makes you more active and alert.

Like the essential oils of most citrus fruits, grapefruit essential oil has an uplifting and relaxing effect on mind. It induces positive feelings of hope, cures depression, and relieves anxiety and stress. This effect comes from two sources. First, due to its aroma, and second, due to its stimulating effects of certain hormones that have uplifting effects on the brain.

Grapefruit essential oil can cause skin irritation if skin is exposed to strong sunlight after application.

Eucalyptus

One very important reason that many people use eucalyptus oil is that it creates a cooling and refreshing effect. Normally, people suffering from certain conditions and disorders are slightly sluggish. Eucalyptus is said to relieve exhaustion and mental sluggishness and rejuvenates the spirits of the sick. It can also be effective in the treatment of stress and mental disorders.

Aside from mental exhaustion, eucalyptus essential oil is commonly used to stimulate mental activity and increase blood flow to the brain. Since the essential oil is considered a vasodilator by many, it means that it increases the blood flow around the body by relaxing the blood vessels and allowing more blood to circulate. Basically, more blood to the brain means more brain power, and eucalyptus essential oil is commonly employed in classrooms as a form of causal aromatherapy to increase student performance. Further formal research must be done in this area, but all signs point to the positive correlation between brain function and eucalyptus essential oil.

If you are experiencing joint and muscle pain, massaging eucalyptus oil on the surface of the skin helps to relieve stress and pain. The versatile eucalyptus oil is analgesic and anti-inflammatory in nature. Therefore, it is often recommended to patients suffering from rheumatism, lumbago, sprained ligaments and tendons, stiff muscles, aches, fibrosis, and even nerve pain. The oil should be massaged in a circular motion on the affected areas of the body.

There are some dangers of taking too much eucalyptus oil, because when taken in large quantities, it can be toxic.

Bergamot

The components of bergamot oil, like alpha-Pinene and limonene, are antidepressant and stimulating in nature. They create a feeling of freshness, joy, and energy in cases of sadness and depression by improving the circulation of the blood.

The flavonoids present in bergamot oil are very good relaxants as well. They soothe nerves and reduce nervous tension, anxiety, and stress, all of which can help cure or treat ailments associated with stress such as sleeplessness, high blood pressure, insomnia, and depression. They can also stimulate the activity of certain hormones like dopamine and serotonin in the body, which induce feelings of relaxation.

Bergamot oil must be protected from sunlight, because bergapten, one of its components, becomes poisonous if exposed to sunlight. That is why the oil should always be stored in dark bottles in dark places. Exposure to sunlight should even be avoided after it is applied or rubbed onto the skin, at least until it absorbs into your skin.

There are of course several other essential oils that you can try out, but these are the ones I mostly commonly use in my own restorative practice and when I teach.

Restorative Through the Lens of Ayurveda

According to Ayurveda—India's ancient healing art and the sister science of yoga—our inner glow or vitality is fueled by *ojas* (pronounced oh-jus), a term that refers to the body's internal energy reserves. *Ojas* energy is described as the end product of good physical and emotional digestion, the result of fully assimilated nutrients and comprehensively processed life experiences.

It's also said to be the essence of *kapha*, the stabilizing water–earth element. Like oil in a lamp, *ojas* sustains our fierier physical and mental energy, our drive and passion. When replenished regularly, *ojas* manifests outwardly in glowing skin, bright eyes, and silky hair. Inwardly, it helps your reproductive, nervous, and immune systems thrive and promotes peaceful emotions such as gratitude and contentment. Most importantly, *ojas* supports stable moods and helps us handle stress with grace and ease. To help cultivate your *ojas*, Ayurveda offers these simple yet powerful tips for letting your inner radiance shine through.

Relaxation and quiet time replenish *ojas*, so making time to give your senses a rest can help maintain your vital beauty. The practice of silence builds your ability for self-reflection, to start to notice the thoughts and emotions and desires that come up without reacting to them.

If you have more of a so-called *vata* imbalance (stress, tension, crashing joints, constipation, anxiety, etc.) then I suggest you start with some gentle flow yoga sequences before taking on restorative yoga, perhaps with a twenty-minute flow, as Mona always instructs for this condition. Something else that works beautifully on a stress imbalance is long, deep breathing, adding visualizations like *sa-hum kriya* (as explained on p. 60) to balance the mind, and also applying essential oils like bergamot or lavender on your wrists and temples in the poses.

For a *pitta* imbalance (inflammation, emotion, anger, irritation, control, headaches, etc.), a walk in nature is phenomenal as well as some gentle weight training. In yoga, focusing on even breaths when in poses and a gentle flow can benefit this condition nicely before restorative poses. In terms of essential oils, the citrus oils and bergamot can be very soothing for a controlling mind.

For a *kapha* imbalance (lethargy, excess fluids in the body, heaviness, melancholy, bitterness, sinus issues, etc.), start with some sweet restorative holds, then follow with some flow at the end. And in terms of essential oils, try eucalyptus or peppermint oils to balance.

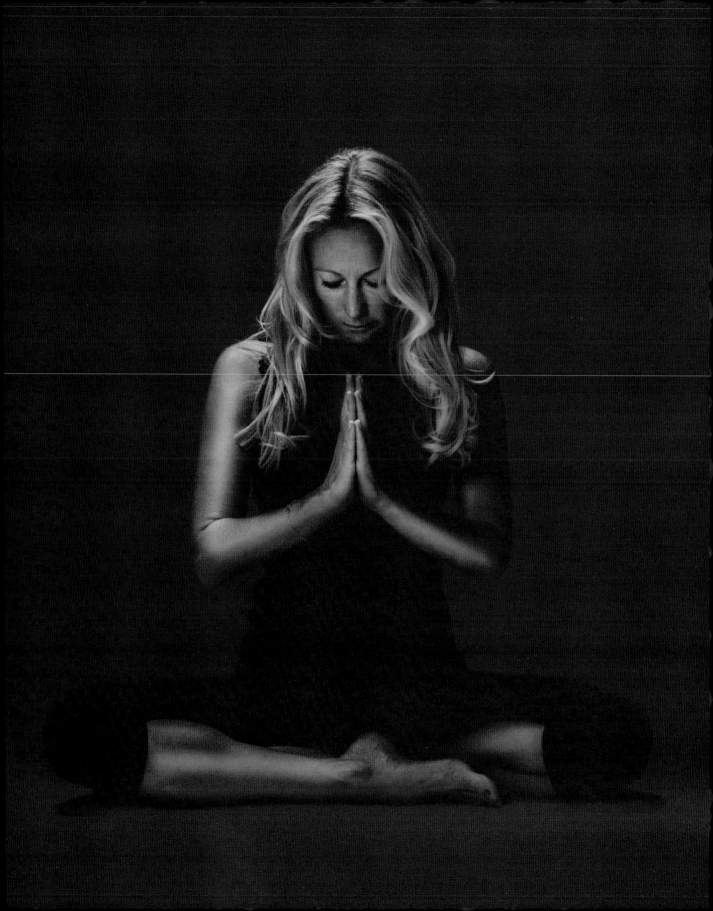

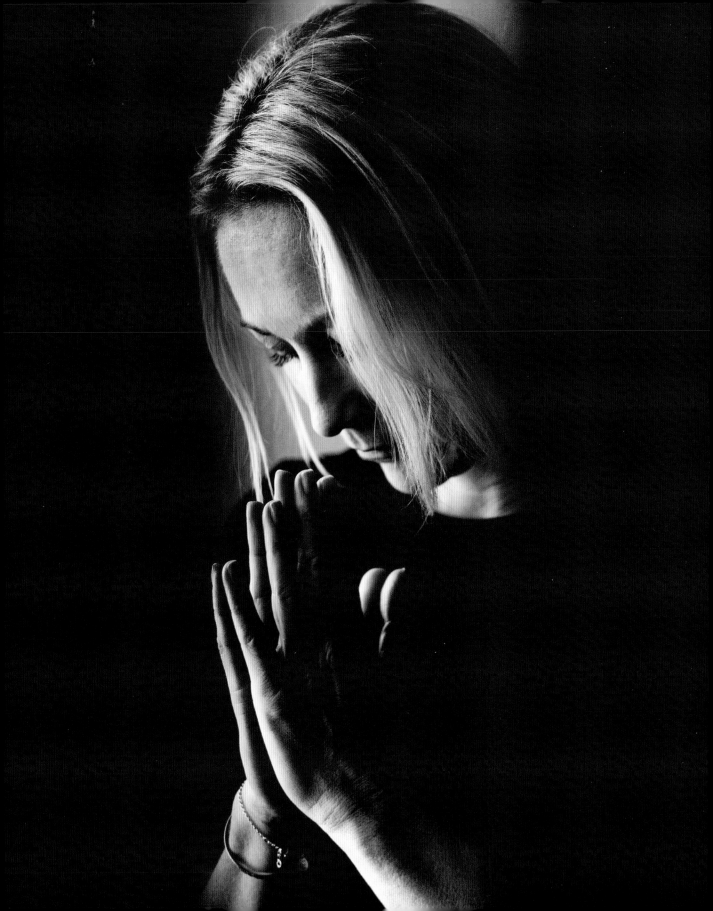

Chapter Five
MEDITATIONS FROM THE MAT

"Rule your mind or it will rule you."
—Buddha

If attaining peace of mind were as simple as reminding ourselves to relax whenever we feel agitated, the majority of us would be blissed-out most of the time. Like any other worthwhile skill, though, relaxation takes practice.

Thankfully, yoga can be a good training ground for cultivating this fine art. And the skills we learn in our yoga practice can support us in the rest of our lives, helping us manage stressful times with clarity and balance.

What can we do to deepen our ability to drop into a state of relaxation and ease? How can we connect with our inner state of peace when our outer lives are awash in stress and chaos? How can we start to make our way back into a better balance in mind, body, spirit, and life?

On and Off the Mat

These suggestions can help you make your way back to balance and tranquility and draw up new pathways toward better relaxation on and off the mat.

EXHALE
One of the best ways to bring yourself back down to earth is to lengthen your exhalations. Include this in your practice, while you transition yourself from one place to another (traveling), when you need to concentrate, focus, and gain inner strength.

This form of breathing—as prescribed in the ancient text *The Yoga Sutras of Patanjali* by Patanjali—encourages the nervous system to become calm and quiet, moving the body into a more restful state of being, more relaxed, and more focused.

INHALE
Some days when you feel sluggish, tired, bored, lethargic, and heavy, just adding some more length to your inhalations might be the ignition toward feeling more alert and awake. In your

yoga practice, start an inhalation softly and gently, and as the inhalation proceeds, increase the effort as you inhale more and more. You do not want to force the breath—you want to feel your ribcage expand and stretch to the fullest, but slowly. Imagine you are breathing with some resistance; keep your mouth closed and visualize drawing in the breath via the nostrils. You want to pull the breath down into yourself, like when you sigh, but with your mouth closed.

FOCUS YOUR MIND

Sometimes when the world sends us spinning, we want to do nothing more than drop into an easy chair and stare into space. But this approach often gives the brain free rein to continue its obsessive and agitated thinking. Instead, try focusing your mind in a constructive and engaging way.

Practice an absorbing breathing exercise, or even simpler than that, stand in *vrksasana* (tree pose) on your right leg (with the left foot on the inside of the right thigh or calf) focus your *drishti* (focal point) on a point in front of you, soften your eyes, face, and jaw, and take 5–10 deep breaths. Repeat on the other leg.

MENTAL DETOX

Try minimizing external stimulation. Turn off the television, unplug the telephone, put the iPads and computers away, and dim the lights. Turn down the volume of your life, remembering that outer calm nurtures inner calm. During your yoga session, use an eye bag or eye wrap while you're in restorative postures to quiet the eyes and the brain. You can also put a heavy bolster on the hips or belly to really unwind when resting in *savasana*. Sometimes we need to really unwind, and if you feel restlessness while in *savasana*, you can try *advasana*—lying on your belly instead with head toward one side. Then breathe into the belly. This is a superior pose for calming down a stressed and restless mind.

SUBSTITUTE POSITIVE THOUGHTS FOR NEGATIVE ONES

The ancient yogic sage Patanjali counseled that when we are disturbed by negative thought patterns, we can recover our balance by inviting peaceful thoughts into our minds. So the next time you find yourself reeling with an agonizing fear or a depressing thought, notice the negative habit, toss it out, and use your creativity to develop a more positive outlook on the world.

When I catch myself thinking negatively about myself, or anything, for that matter, I start a list of what I have in my life that works—of people I like, of great memories, things I have so much to be grateful for (that my toes can move, I can breathe, I am actually alive on this earth right now), of the things I have in my life that I love. Try doing the same, and don't stop until a smile appears on your face. Then you will see that all that negative junk is superfluous.

FEEDING NEW HABITS

Look at your agenda, or your calendar. From a distance. Our outlook on life is a direct reflection of how we perceive ourselves. Where and when do you nurture your ability to be, see beyond the given, to learn more about your inner you, and when do you actually restore your energies?

Start feeding new habits. Good ones that resonate with you on all levels. One example is taking twenty minutes up to an hour (whatever you feel you can fit in) where you don't *do* anything. A moment free from any kind of dialogue, even with yourself. Just observing. Just trying to be with what is. Make space.

Ask yourself: Do you give yourself any space in between things you plan throughout the day? Do you give yourself a proper lunch break?

"You" time. Weekly. Now. Go.

SEEK OUT LAUGHTER

There's nothing more stress-busting than a first-class belly laugh. Call your funniest friend, rent a comedy on video, or attempt a complicated arm balance that will likely leave you swaying and splattering to the floor.

GO OUT IN NATURE

Play in the fall leaves, make snow angels in the snow, take a long walk, walk barefoot in the sand on a beach, go for a hike, lay down in the grass in the summer and just look at clouds. Feel how the ground and earth holds on to you, holds you. Just melt into the earth.

Best restorative yoga ever.

TRY SELF LOVE

There's nothing more stress-busting than a first-class belly laugh. Call your friend that always makes you laugh, watch a stand up comedy act live or on TV or just play Twister with your friends or family—something that makes you not take yourself so seriously. Laughing releases a lot of tension.

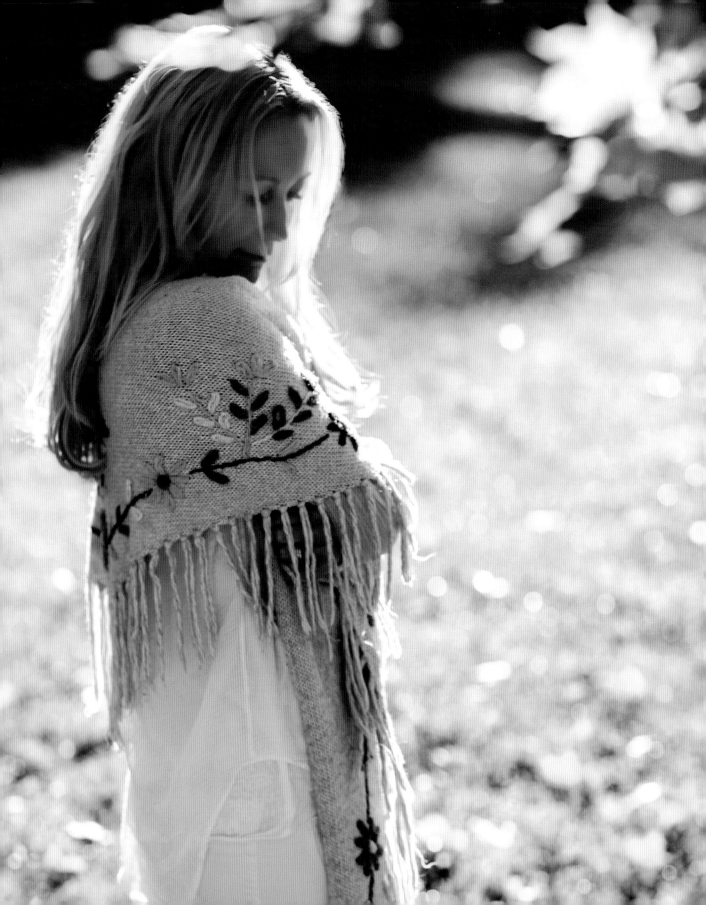

Self love is about supporting yourself in who you are now. It is the foundation that you stand on to create yourself and your life. Your personal power is intimately connected with your foundation of unconditional love. If you can't find unconditional love within and instead you look for it outside of yourself, then your personal power will always follow that seeking—meaning that you will always be giving away your power to those who agree to love you.

One day I woke up with an idea: here we are, celebrating birthdays, successes, weddings, births, etc. But why don't we just give ourselves a Self-Celebration Day? I thought about it, then threw that idea away, thinking it was lame, selfish, and stupid. But the idea lingered with me for a year or two.

Then, last year (2015) on September 21 (International Peace Day), I decided to do it anyway. To give myself a day where I celebrated my life, just being alive, doing my best with what I have and know, and all the efforts made to be my own best friend. I took the day off and just planned things I loved doing. And I was very particular that I spent time alone and with people I really love. It was the scariest day for me. It left me thinking why don't we do this for all of us? Why should we be ashamed of celebrating our own existence? This day not only left a big smile on my face, it brought so much inner joy and tears of gratitude for allowing myself to be and feel nurtured and also for focusing on things that really matter. Did I feel calm, restored, and in better balance?

YES.

So I have decided to mark a day in the calendar each year to do this. I have decided to make March 10 my celebration day. Why that day? Just because I like March and I like the number 10.

Try it for yourself!

PRACTICE, PRACTICE, PRACTICE

Like fine wine, relaxation improves over time. Even if you don't happen to feel completely blissed-out in *savasana* today, you are priming the body for quiet and ease tomorrow. Repeatedly practicing restful postures greases the wheel of relaxation, so you will be able to quickly and easily drop into a deep state of ease someday in the future.

To create the right atmosphere for restorative yoga, start by choosing a comfortable, warm, quiet, and safe place. Keep it quite dark, maybe with some candles burning to give a soothing ambiance to the room.

According to Gina, "the dark setting triggers sleep stimulators and if you use the eye pillow, it will help induce the relaxation response in the brain. Be mindful to cover the hands and feet since the warmth will help you to relax and unwind mentally. Also, start to lie in some poses for longer times since the stretch reflex in muscles takes time to release, and the neurotransmitters that kick in from the fight or flight response take longer to break down through chemical processing than does the neurotransmitter that kicks in from the relaxation response."[5]

Start every pose with even, long breaths, starting to surrender into your props, feeling that you can float in the pose, that nothing feels like it is interfering with you. Don't feel any stretch in the poses, just yummy-ness. Then just breathe yourself into the pose, and bathe in some floating state.

One thing that sometimes helps me is calm, soothing music in the background. Or, just listening to my breath. If I do it outside, when the weather allows, feeling the breeze on my face and sounds of nature can be a part of my experience.

Restorative Yoga in Combination with Sports

Getting into a flow mindset (often described as being "in the zone") can help athletes to consistently achieve optimal performance. Flow is often defined as a mental state in which the individual transcends conscious thought and achieves a heightened state of effortless and unwavering concentration, calm, and confidence. This flow state keeps pressures and distractions, both internal and external, from creeping into athletes' minds and potentially harming their performance.

Athletes who can achieve, maintain, and regain flow are mentally tough, and the ability to do this is critical for achieving personal excellence in sports. Restorative yoga for athletes helps them to drain toxins out of the muscles, to mentally unwind, and to reduce tension in mind

---

5. See *Anand Menza Restorative Training Manual*:
Mona Anand, Gina Menza, ISHTA Yoga
New York, New York 2012.

and body. This not only balances their bodies, but increases their mental capacity to focus even when challenged. Restorative yoga also helps athletes remain injury-free; when injured, restorative yoga is a phenomenal tool that helps to increase healing in the tissues, especially in the fascia.

I have the privilege to coach professional athletes in yoga and meditation and we work with different techniques depending on who they are, where they are in life, what sport they perform, and what they need to enhance in order to better their performances. I have worked with some professional cross country skiers, track and fielders, soccer players, hockey players, gymnasts, boxers, snow boarders, and ballerinas. And with many of them, I introduce restorative yoga as a means to restore, reboot, rebuild, and de-stress the body, mind, and soul. At first they were skeptical, but after only a couple of sessions, they loved it and felt it was so easy to bring with them on tours and camps. Several of them have actually claimed that they are much more focused, more poised, don't get injured as easily, that their bodies respond to the other training they do, and they achieve better results and feel better about themselves and what they do. One of the soccer players said that he was able to heal a severe calf injury so much faster than he ever thought possible just with the practice I gave him.

This reinforces in me that this practice has so much intelligence in it since it allows us to reconnect back to ourselves, to unwind the busyness our minds are wound up in. When the mind quiets, then the body gets stronger.

A flow state isn't just helpful for athletes. Surgeons performing challenging, state-of-the-art procedures report experiencing intense flow comparable to pro athletes. But flow states can also occur when we're writing, dancing, cooking, or even reading a book. It helps us to become deeply involved with anything we're doing, and many times is the secret to a more joyful life.

It is the full involvement of flow, rather than happiness, that makes for excellence in life. We can be happy experiencing the passive pleasure of a rested body, warm sunshine, or the contentment of a serene relationship, but this kind of happiness is dependent on favorable external circumstances. The happiness that follows flow is of our own making, and it leads to increasing complexity and growth in consciousness.

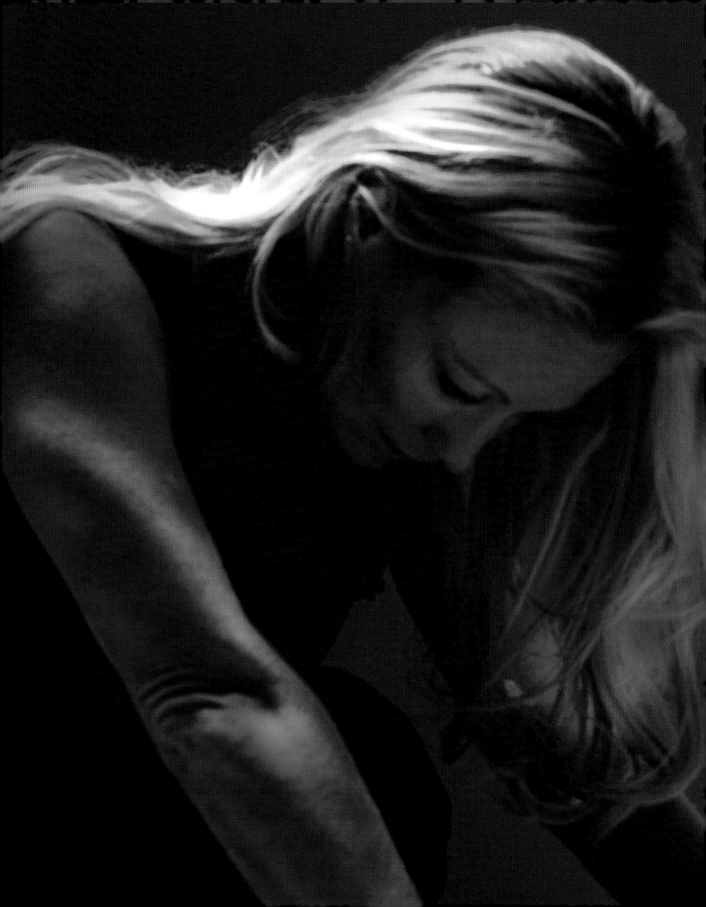

The powers we seek are in the pauses. Within the pauses, when we reflect, when the body calibrates, is where magic happens. That is where our inner forces can be grasped.

We are often so busy looking back and forth in life that we become weak in pausing, reflecting, and noticing the details around and within ourselves. Restorative yoga is about rediscovering the known—regularly.

Restorative Yoga and Coming Out of Exhaustion and Depression

When it comes to depression and how to use yoga as a remedy to slowly build up more energy and come back from exhaustion, let's revisit the *gunas* one more time. As with all imbalances in us, we are under the influence of *rajas* and *tamas* and, according to yogic philosophy, we need to balance these two aspects in order to attain better energy and balance.

Tamas is linked to the earth element. It is associated with steadiness and stability, calming hormones as well as inertia, poor circulation, and sluggishness. *Rajas* is associated with activity, adrenaline, doing, and action as well as greed and restlessness. *Sattva* is associated with balance in the nervous system, mental clarity, peace, and the pursuit of spiritual activities.

According to this framework, the nature of depression depends on which of these qualities is dominant. Yoga postures are selected based on their ability to counteract or correct these (*tamasic* or *rajasic*) imbalances.

A person with a depression dominated by *tamas* may experience fatigue, lethargy, and hopelessness. Their posture tends to be collapsed and their shoulders turned inward. Yoga poses that open the chest and shoulders and facilitate deeper breathing can help to provide physical and energetic relief and increase the flow of *prana*, or upward energy. In restorative, a pose like *supta baddha konasana* can be a marvelous pose to do twenty minutes, 4–5 times a week.

Unlike the dullness of *tamasic* depression, *rajasic*-dominated symptoms of depression include anxiety, restlessness, and agitation along with depressed mood. Restorative yoga postures that make use of forward bends are believed to activate parasympathetic nervous system (PNS) activity and to provide some relief. Here, a supported child's pose and also a gentle inversion like *viparita karani* for ten minutes every day can work wonders.

The overall aim when practicing yoga to relieve depression is to increase the quality of *sattva* in our cognitive-emotional make-up. So, in restorative yoga, keeping a balanced practice is a smart thing to do. That can mean doing a twenty-minute pose each night before bed or when in need during the day, but have different days involve different poses. So, in a week you would complete a restorative sequence. And once a month, take ninety minutes to do one of the longer sequences, and bring the poses together in one go.

Sattva is associated with life-supporting qualities and feelings of lightness, happiness, and well-being. Following this principle, the foods we eat can also impact our well-being. Staying away from heavy, processed, hard-to-digest foods and emphasizing foods with a more nourishing quality like fruits, vegetables, and whole grains can also help support the healing process.

Our understanding of how yoga can help relieve depression is still in its infancy, and it's important to keep in mind that depression can be a serious condition. Take it on slowly.

Since I have suffered from exhaustion myself, I know a little bit of what I am talking about. For me, when I was totally drained, everything that involved strong movements would get my heart racing and I would feel sad, vulnerable, and just wanted to sleep and not take any part in the outside world. I hated emails, I cringed when someone would call me, and said no to all social invitations. I withdrew as much as I could.

Thank God for my husband and kids being there for me and forcing me to come out of my shell from time to time. Also, my teacher, Alan Finger, guided me in my practice and gave me things to work on that were not too demanding. Gentle moving, *pranayama*/breathing exercises, and short meditation was all I could do. And sometimes some short walks outside, though occasionally that, too, was too much for me. It took me almost a year to get back to a better balance, and I don't know how long it would have taken without the tools I had. Slowly I added more time in restorative poses, I could sit longer in yin yoga poses and my walks became slightly longer.

I am always of aware of my depression and I have to be mindful of my energies and balance all I have on my plate wisely in order not to get exhausted. I am a person with a passion for living and life and I want to create, be, do, and be a part of my outside world. So I use the Full Complete Breath (as described on page 35) a lot: I balance every strong activity or strenuous working day with some down time and gentle yoga.

Another thing worth mentioning is that after one comes out of a period of exhaustion and depression, the body carries more excess tension and excess toxins that need to come out. So combining restorative yoga with some gentle weight training, maybe jogging and flowing yoga, is a great way of detoxifying and de-stressing. Also, I cannot stress enough going out in nature as much as one can—being in its silence and natural sounds, walking, hiking, or just sitting and watching its splendor. Let Nature's arms catch and hold you and help you shed layers of stress and tension. Put on the brakes in your life, break out from urban living for a while. It will save your life.

Life is a roller coaster between highs and lows. We all know that, have felt it, tasted it, experienced it, and picked our own brains on how and why in order to understand, fix, nuance it or just try to cope with life as it is.

We don't usually stop and reflect over our lives when life is good to us and when we are in a high.

However, it is when we get hurt, hit a bump, feel betrayed, traumatized, get questioned, come into a crisis, or just don't get our way with things, that we stop and look up—and often react to it with emotions. And then we hurt more and go deeper into that negativity.

Yogic philosophy inspires us to quiet our minds, strengthen our bodies, and see beyond the limitations of mind and emotional reactions. When our consciousness is not so clouded by reactions we can really be alive, aware, strong, and present.

What we perceive as real or the truth—what is that truth made of and who and what gives us that truth? Yoga and meditation offer tools to inquire of yourself and the world in order to see things more clearly and connect to your own and universal intelligence. When we release loads of tension that haunt our bodies and minds, we open our hearts and then we are able to be present, aware, and loving.

I have spent over twenty years personally inquiring of my inside and my outside, trying to find out who I am and what resonates with me, and to find ways to balance my strengths with my limitations.

What this investment has given me is proof of the following: when we are stuck in our minds and in the past, in the limitations, we are inhibiting our potential to heal from coming forth. Life is always going to present challenges to you.

In my teens, some people called me a boundless searcher with an empty intention. "Nothing good will come out of that search, you will only be more lost." Others have called after me, "You are wasting your talents," and there have been voices of those feeling that I do too much, am too much, feel too much—that I am just being too much.

To some extent they have been right. I have felt lost at times. And I have been too much. And not enough. But that part about having no intention—there, I don´t agree. My intention has always been about the aphorism "Know thyself." This quest means in being lost you find something.

So thank you, all who have critiqued and praised me, because that has helped me to stay on my path. Still exploring the unbound potential of my individuality, understanding that I am not only my personality. Your comments and actions have made me stronger and clearer. Today.

I have always had this inner voice saying to me to trust the path and all that is happening. To trust the fact that there is a *Self* to be known. *My* Self. That has kept me going.

Often I ponder where I got the energy to move forward. Well, I guess part is a heritage from my ancestors and family, many of whom are fighters and strong individual people. Part is from influence and exposure to great self-balancing (yoga and meditation), inspiring people, ideas, different cultures, movements, nature, books, and music.

My path has led me to not fear myself. To look beyond the given and take it from there. To go inside and connect to spirit. Spirit is one's existence, the underlying connection to life and what is beyond. We can think of spirituality as our connection to life, to creation, to our existence.

I know from my own experience that there is a lot of fear related to the aspect of spirit. I think it has a lot to do with us leading our lives according to rules, socialized norms, and values not created by ourselves but from dogma of certain types. If we have a weak relationship to ourselves, we seek meaning in religion or science. In science, where only reason counts as truth, and religion where dogmatic rules set a way of living, equal for all.

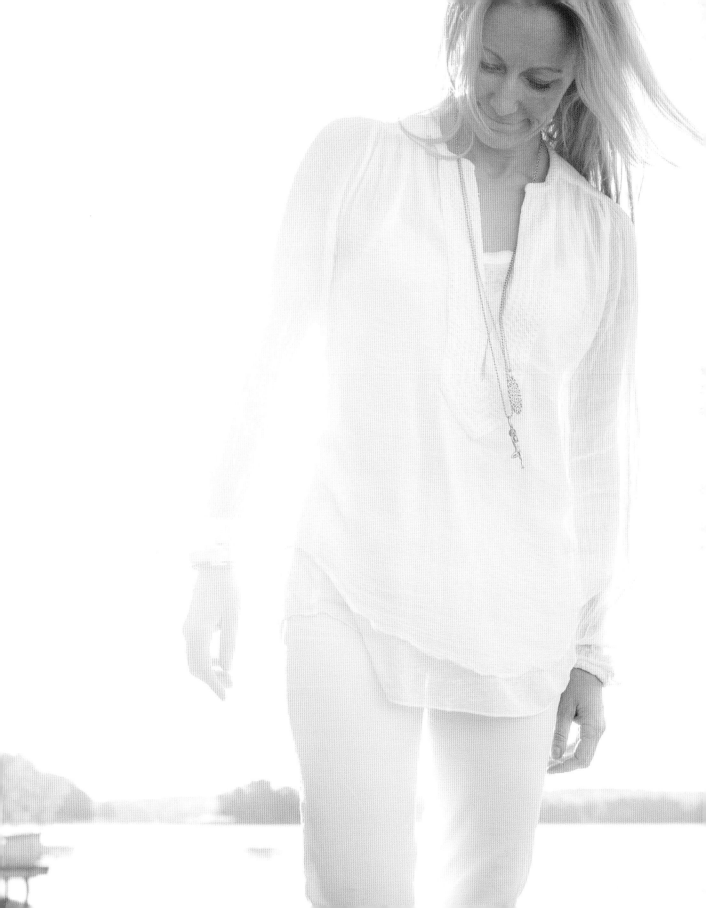

Spirituality extends beyond an expression of religion or practice of religion. There is a pursuit for a spiritual dimension that not only inspires but creates harmony with the universe. That relationship between ourselves and something greater compels us to seek answers about the infinite.

During times of intense emotional, mental, or physical stress, man searches for transcendent meaning, oftentimes through music, nature, arts, or a set of philosophical beliefs. This often results in a broad set of principles that transcends all religions and science.

The search for spirituality and meaning, man's connection to something beyond the temporal, sends him/her down paths that offer unsatisfactory results.

My life journey has shown me that transparency is one interesting way to move forward. In order to attain more transparency in life, we need to reduce tension and look into our inner darkness. Ask questions, be scientific and do research, but also stop and just be with what is, in order to connect to aspects that we do not yet know or see in front of us, but lie within us. How do we do that? Well, I think the yogic tradition is on to something, believing that spirit and science can go hand in hand to help us reach our inner potential as individuals and as a whole.

When you start taking yourself too seriously, the yoga is gone. This practice is all about investigation and exploration in order for light and insight to appear.

Restorative yoga, conscious breathing, and meditation are certainly things that have elevated not only my life to heights I never thought possible, but also healed many inner and external wounds while helping me to become incredibly strong mentally, emotionally, spiritually, and physically—beyond what I thought was possible.

I hope this book has inspired you to begin to explore this practice on your own and together with inspiring teachers, and hopefully attain tools to start to build a more transparent, stress-reduced, loving, clear, interesting, and strong life.

Jai ma,

Ulrica

STOCKHOLM, January 2016

REFERENCES

Restorative Yoga:

Anand Menza Restorative Training Manual: Mona Anand, Gina Menza, ISHTA Yoga. New York, New York 2012

Amygdala and Changes:

Britta K. Hölzel, James Carmody, Karleyton C. Evans, Elizabeth A. Hoge, Jeffery A. Dusek, Lucas Morgan, Roger K. Pitman and Sara W. Lazar. 2009 "Stress Reduction Correlates with Structural Changes in the Amygdala." *Oxford Journals* 5(1): 11-17. doi: 10.1093/scan/nsp034.

Meditation and ANS control:

Sara W. Lazar, George Bush, Randy L. Gollub, Gregory L. Fricchione, Gurucharan Khalsa, and Herbert Benson. 2000. "Functional Brain Mapping of the Relaxation Response and Meditation." *NeuroReport* 11(7): 1581-1585. doi: 10.1097/00001756-200005150-00041.

Hebbs Law:

Hebb, D.O. 1949. *The Organization of Behavior*. New York: Wiley & Sons.

Neurogenesis:

Kirsty L. Spalding, Olaf Bergmann, Kanar Alkass, Samuel Bernard, Mehran Salehpour, Hagen B. Huttner, Emil Boström, Isabelle Westerlund, Celine Vial, Bruce A. Buchholz, Göran Possnert, Deborah C. Mash, Henrik Druid, and Jonas Frisén. 2016. "Dynamics of Hippocampal Neurogenesis in Adult Humans." *PMC* doi: 10.1016/j.cell.2013.05.002.

Cognitive Change from Meditation:

Cortland J. Dahl, Antoine Lutz, Richard J. Davidson. 2015. "Reconstructing and Deconstructing the Self: Cognitive Mechanisms in Meditation Practice." *Trends in Cognitive Sciences* doi: 10.1016/j.tics.2015.07.001.

R. Davidson and A. Kaszniak. 2015. "Conceptual and Methodological Issues in Research on Mindfulness and Meditation." *American Psychologist* doi: 10.1037/a0039512.

Davidson and B. S. Schuyler. 2015. Neuroscience of Happiness. In *World Happiness*, edited by J.F. Helliwell, R. Layard, and J. Sachs, chapter 5. New York: The Earth Institute, Columbia University.

Mindfulness and Neurogenesis:

Britta K. Hölzel, James Carmody, Mark Vangel, Christina Congleton, Sita M. Yerramsetti, Tim Gard, and Sara W. Lazar. 2011. "Mindfulness Practice Leads to Increases in Regional Brain Gray Matter Density." *Psychiatry Research* doi: 10.1016/j.pscychresns.2010.08.006.

Tensegrity:
Donald E. Ingber. 2003. "Tensegrity I. Cell Structure and Hierarchical Systems of Biology." *Journal of Cell Science* doi: 10.1242/jcs.00359.

Sherri Cassuto. 2012. "Thoughts on Tensegrity and Hydrostatics in Human Architecture." *Structural Integration.*

Hypnogogic State:
Michael Samuels and Nancy Samuels. 1975. *Seeing with the Mind´s Eye.* New York: Random House.

Andreas Mavromatis. 1987. *Hypnagogia: The Unique State of Consciousness Between Wakefulness and Sleep.* London: Routledge.

Relaxation Response:
Herbert Benson and Miriam Klipper. 1974. *The Relaxation Response.* New York: Taylor and Francis.

Neuroplasticity:
Bogdan Draganski, Christian Gaser, Volker Busch, Gerhard Schuierer, Ulrich Bogdahn, and Arne May 2004. "Neuroplasticity: Changes in Grey Matter Induced by Training." *Nature* doi: 10.1038/427311a.

B.S. McEwen. 2012. "The Ever-changing Brain: Cellular and Molecular Mechanisms for the Effects of Stressful Experiences." *Developmental Neurobiology* doi: 10.1002/dneu.20968.

Norman Doidge, MD. 2007. *The Brain That Changes Itself.* New York: Penguin Books.

Code:
Erwin Schrödinger. 1944. *What is Life.* Cambridge: Cambridge University Press.

Sleep:
Roger Cole. 2005. "Nonpharmacologic Techniques for Promoting Sleep." *Clinics in Sports Medicine* doi:10.1016/j.csm.2004.12.010.

ACKNOWLEDGMENTS

Every time I sit down to write my thanks, I think it is the last opportunity I'll have to write a book and I worry about missing someone. I fear I am in the wrong mindset to transparently list all who have helped me with this book process.

There are so many people and so many things that have impacted my life. From family, animals, teachers, colleagues, friends, and authors, to travels, movies I have seen, and moments on my yoga mat all alone.

In writing a book, so many aspects of oneself come out and are used and reused and molded in various ways. So where does one start?

After stopping, pausing, and breathing, I ponder and meditate on this for a while, and somewhat clearer nuances emerge.

I wish to thank myself for giving me time, moments, and encounters with silence and stillness and also for challenging myself physically, emotionally, and mentally. I guess that sounds weird, but I feel I would never have written this book if it wasn't for my open mind, daring soul, and curious being. I also want to thank my inner darkness, my destructive moments, and all those not so enlightened situations in my life.

I want to thank life. Thank you for showing me the highs and the lows, for giving me so many situations to grow from, and showing me so many aspects of thinking, feeling, living, moving, and being.

When it comes to certain individuals that have supported me throughout this process, I first and foremost wish to thank my family: my husband and best friend who has stood by my side through every book, including this one. And my children for being there, giving me space and so much love. I am amazed at how much they "get" even though they are such small children. They teach me so much. I love you *so* much.

Thank you also to:

Hillevi Borga, MSC and PhT, my dear friend and colleague for making time to be interviewed and for sharing your wealth of knowledge. It is so lovely to have a friend who shares my passion for yoga, meditation, spirituality, and science.

Cecilia Duberg, Cert. Psychologist, for your time and generosity with sharing your knowledge and for your passion for humanity, personal growth, science, and resarch.

Bengt Ljungquist, PhD in Neuroscience at Lunds University, for your friendship, intelligence, passion, and drive. Without people like you there would be no building bridges between different worlds. And that is the future.

Mona Anand, Yogiraj (Yogamaster) in ISHTA yoga, restorative/Yoga Nidra specialist, you are such a soul sister who I love dearly and I love working with you as well as learning from you. Just being who you are is guidance for so many around you.

Gina Menza, Senior ISHTA yoga teacher, you are such a smart, witty, and lovely human being, woman, and friend. Being around you always brings joy and love into my heart and smiles to my face. And sharing the passion for the stillness in yoga with you is phenomenal to me.

Judith Hanson Lasater, PhT and restorative yoga expert, you mean so much to the yoga community. Thanks to your guidance and dedication to this practice, you have shown so many people the path to restoration of one's energies in such classy, smart ways. Thank you for being you.

Kavi Yogi Alan Finger, my dear teacher, mentor, and friend. Thank you for supporting me and for being a lightbearing and guiding spirit in my personal growth and progression as a human being, yogi, and teacher. Your prescence is so dear to me and has made such a difference in my life. Thank you for all your kindness and for contributing to this book through interviews, support, and sources of information.

Clas von Sydow, journalist, dear teacher and now friend. You made such an impression on me with your tireless, passionate interest for the human sciences, your phenomenal teaching skills, and super inspiring ways. Thank you for guiding me to be better. Thank you for making hard work be so rewarding.

Sebastian Forsman for excellent teamwork with the photographs, Abigail Gehring and crew at Skyhorse Publishing in New York City for once again believing in what I have to share.

And special thanks to Johan and Nyström, my local café, for being such a heartful and warm hangout, and to all my students and readers for all of your support.

Without you I wouldn´t be here. THANK YOU!

Namaste,

Ulrica

ABOUT THE AUTHOR

Ulrica Norberg has been studying and teaching yoga for over twenty-five years and has extensive experience in a wide range of different yogic systems. Her teaching style is knowledgeable, inspirational, generous, and warm and reflects elements from her own meditation and yoga practice, teaching experience, life, and studies. She has a Master's degree in film and journalism, lived in the US for many years, and traveled immensely around the world before returning to her native Sweden, where she lives today with her husband and their two children.

Since the nineties, Ulrica has played an important role in yoga's growth in Europe. She has trained over five hundred yoga teachers and is an admired teacher, trainer, and mentor, and is the author of several articles, books, and films on yoga.

Today, Ulrica works as a dramatist, editor, and writer as well as lecturer and coach for individuals, athletes, and organizations, and teaches yoga and meditation trainings, retreats, and workshops in Scandinavia, Europe, and in the US. In Spring of 2015, she reached the highest honor a yogi can receive in modern time when she was initiated to Yoga Master (Yogiraj) by Kavi Yogi Alan Finger, which makes her the first Scandinavian to reach such a level of achievement in yoga.

WEBSITE:
www.ulricanorberg.se
Instagram: ulricanorberg
Twitter: ulricanorberg